Creative Puppetry

with Children & Adults

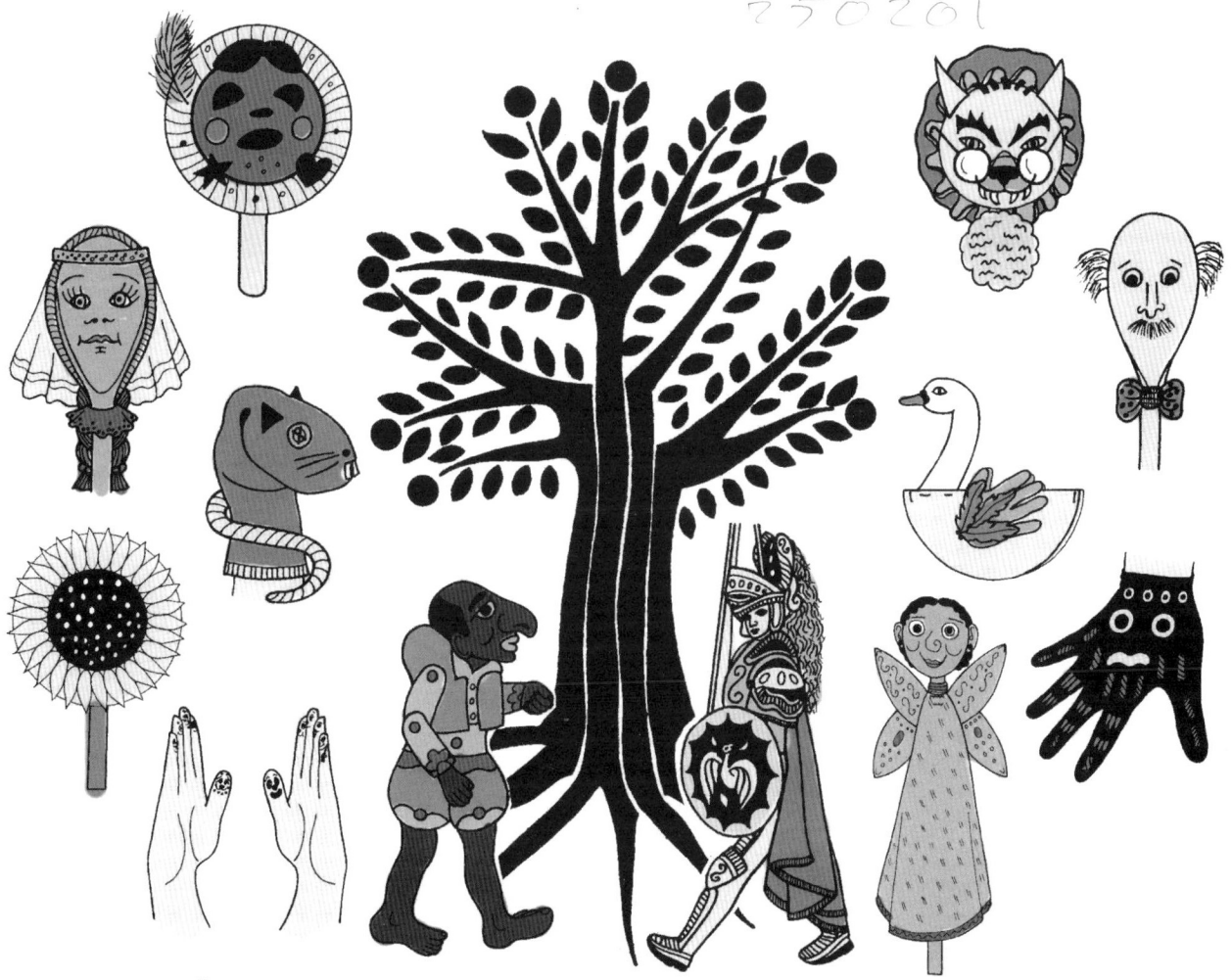

Sue Jennings

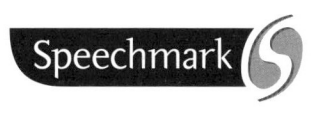
Speechmark

I am dedicating this book to my youngest grandchildren:
Leon, Mir, Kaia and Mary.
They have all inspired me to tell stories and play with puppets.

Cover design and all illustrations by Suzanne Hall.

First published in 2008 by
Speechmark Publishing Ltd, 70 Alston Drive, Bradwell Abbey, Milton Keynes, MK13 9HG, United Kingdom
Tel: +44 (0) 1908 326942   Fax: +44 (0) 1908 326958
www.speechmark.net

002-5373/Printed in the United Kingdom/1010

British Library Cataloguing in Publication Data
Jennings, Sue, 1938–
        Creative puppetry with children & adults
        1. Puppets – Therapeutic use
        I. Title
        616.8'91653

ISBN: 978 0 86388 609 6

Contents

List of Worksheets   v

Acknowledgements   vii

Introduction   1

Chapter 1:   **Why Puppets? A Short History**   5

Chapter 2:   **Fun with Fingers**   14
Simple finger puppets and how to make them

Chapter 3:   **Simple Dolls and Puppets**   32

Chapter 4:   **Hands as Puppets**   51

Chapter 5:   **Stick Puppets – A Stick is not just a Stick**   68

Chapter 6:   **Shadow Puppets**   85

Chapter 7:   **Puppets on Poles – Larger than Life**   104

Chapter 8:   **Puppets with Mouth**   128
Ready-made puppets for therapy and education; generational puppets; animal hand and sleeve puppets; how to make a moving mouth animal and person

Chapter 9:   **Story Dolls: Evoking Stories**   149
Story Dolls for storytelling: water, earth, fire and air; old myths and legends. How to make Story Dolls

Chapter 10:   **Good Yarns for Puppets and Dolls**   172

Chapter 11:   **Useful Addresses**   189

Chapter 12:   **Bibliography**   196

List of Worksheets

Chapter 2

2.1	Fingers as Puppets	22
2.2	Spider Puppets	24
2.3	Simple Finger Puppets	26
2.4	Fabric Finger Puppets	28
2.5	Easy-Peasy Puppets	30

Chapter 3

3.1	Cotton Glove Puppet	45
3.2	Feelings Doll	47
3.3	Simple Story Doll	49

Chapter 4

4.1	Spider Glove Puppets	64
4.2	Rat Sock Puppet	65
4.3	Moving Mouth Sock Puppets	66
4.4	Creating Stories for your Puppets	67

Chapter 5

5.1	The Story of the Thunder Bird	83
5.2	The Birth of Athena – A Stick Puppet Play	84

Chapter 6

6.1	The Story of the Poisoned Apple	93
6.2	Greek Shadow Puppets – Karaghiozis	98
6.3	Greek Shadow Puppets – Baba Yiorgos	99
6.4	Scenario between Karaghiozis and Baba Yiorgos	100
6.5	Greek Shadow Puppets – Morfonios	101
6.6	Greek Shadow Puppets – Sir Dionysios	103

Chapter 7

7.1	Puppets on Poles – Red Riding Hood	124
7.2	Puppets for The Children of Lir	125
7.3	The Children of Lir – creating a Swan Puppet	126
7.4	The Children of Lir – alternative Swan Puppet	127

Chapter 8

8.1	Simple Person Puppet	145
8.2	Simple Animal Puppet	147

Chapter 9

9.1	Making a Mermaid Story Doll	166
9.2	Making a Silkie Story Doll	168
9.3	Making a Story Doll with Legs	170

Acknowledgements

FAMILY AND FRIENDS HAVE HELPED enormously with the writing of this book, especially Aanand Chabukswar. I would like to thank Sharon Jacksties and the Storyroots Project, Nicola Grove and The Unlimited Company and the Wells Stroke Group for patience, inspiration and stories. Pauline Royce has helped me with the Story Dolls and continues to make glorious sacred dolls. Gayle Kearney has helped me with the cotton hand puppet. Sue Hall has helped me put the whole project together. Thank you all.

Dr Sue Jennings
Wells, Somerset

Introduction

THIS BOOK DESCRIBES THE PRACTICAL MAKING of puppets that can be a source of delight and exploration for children and adults. Often people want to create a very specific character to express their feelings or tell their stories.

Chapters 2–5 (*Fun with Fingers* to *Stick Puppets* inclusive) are all concerned with the practicalities of making simple finger, glove, shadow and rod puppets that need basic materials. Instructions for making the puppets are given on worksheets at the end of the chapter. Many of these can be made from scraps such as odd gloves or socks. We shall add stories and props and simple puppet and theatre playing space.

The following five chapters describe the use of puppets we may have bought or made before we start work with children or adults and also include many stories for puppet work.

> **Many children will relate to puppets when they are unable to relate to other people. This is particularly the case with children with behavioural and emotional difficulties.**

Using Puppets in a Therapeutic Setting

Puppets can be used for the telling of personal stories. This may be the child's own story or they may tell it through a fairy tale or legend. Puppets, whether individual ones, or a group or a family will allow the child to communicate the complexity of their situation which will often involve divided loyalties. It is rare that the child's situation is unilinear and there will be a complicated time frame in the past, present and future, multiple spaces, and several perceptions both of relationships and events.

Often it will need more than one session and more than one puppet for the child to communicate. The advantage of puppet work is that the child (or adult) has control over the puppets and that it is 'once removed' from the child's (or adults') direct experience.

Puppets can be used for theme-based work such as education in drug abuse or bullying. Students aged 11–16 often want to present issues that are of direct relevance to them, and that concern their day-to-day lives.

Many children will enjoy the creation of a puppet play and presenting it to others. The children can make the puppets and tell the story, either devised from their own ideas or created from a traditional tale. Many children discover that through the puppets they can find a voice of their own, and be heard!

Puppets also have an important place in the transitions that children have to make in their lives, for example when they go to hospital or move house. Puppets are rather like masks that are not directly on the face, and have the same varied properties. Puppets and masks both 'conceal and reveal' and enable the safe exploration of themes and feelings that would otherwise be internalised. Many children are not articulate enough to express their fears and anxieties, and the puppets can facilitate this.

Generally, puppet work is a projective activity but it can also be relevant to all three stages of EPR (Embodiment-Projection-Role) development as I have described in many previous publications (listed in the Bibliography). For example, in embodiment (E), puppets can help children learn about appropriate touch and the way we treat our own bodies as well as other people's bodies. They can demonstrate gestures and movement and can 'model' movement games and playing. They can also represent the senses and feelings. The puppets themselves can be very sensory when touched.

Puppets can be projective (P) characters in games and stories and can undertake projective activities that children may find difficult. For example, the puppet can draw or model or make a puzzle. It can build the bricks and knock them down again. The puppet can in fact become the play worker or teacher's assistant. The puppet can also be the child's friend or confidante.

Puppets can take on any roles (R) that the child or teacher chooses: you may decide to have a puppet each and enter into a dialogue or create a play or share secrets. You may make use of several puppets that are part of the narrative.

Children with special needs often have difficulty in communication and social skills. They may be nervous or shy, or be suffering from neglect. They may have poor concentration or be hyperactive. I find that puppet-making and use can often overcome many of these difficulties. The puppet becomes the focus of the attention and comes to life in so many different ways. The child suddenly exists through this new medium.

Try practising with your puppets before you work with children: it is easy to use a silly voice because you feel nervous! It is a good idea to choose a well-known story and tell the story with your puppet(s) until you feel at ease with them. You are not trying to be a ventriloquist! If you feel confident with a puppet then the child will also feel confident.

Remember that a puppet is really an extension of our own hand – and most of us use our hands expressively, especially when we are telling stories. Above all, puppet work can develop a child's confidence and creativity and enable participation in the wider social world.

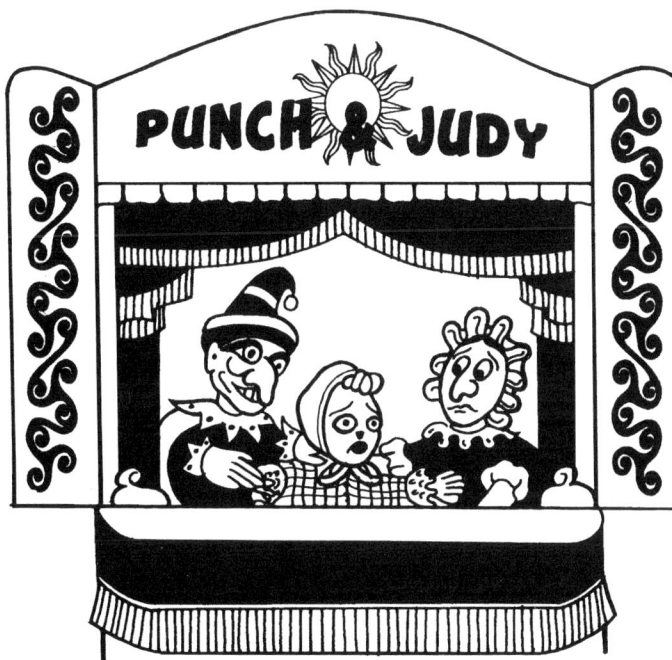

CHAPTER 1

Why Puppets?

Tᴏ ᴛʜᴇ ɪᴍᴘᴏʀᴛᴀɴᴄᴇ ᴏꜰ ᴘᴜᴘᴘᴇᴛꜱ ɪɴ ᴇᴅᴜᴄᴀᴛɪᴏɴ and therapy cannot be over-estimated, and a brief look at its roots will help us to understand why puppets continue to be a powerful means of expression and communication for children and adults alike.

A Short History

Puppets and marionettes feature in many ancient civilisations and reference is made to them in writings of the Greeks and the Romans. Some researchers believe that puppetry began in India some 4,000 years ago with shadow puppets (Dugan, 1990), but it is also suggested that the masks with moveable jaws were the first attempts at animation, and these masks have an even older history. China and Japan all have ancient puppet traditions. More recently puppets have been linked to traditions in Italy and also the former Czechoslovakia. It is thought that the word puppet is linked to the word for doll: *pupa* in Latin, *pupée* in French, for example. Dolls in modern times are separate from puppets; children talk to their dolls and then sometimes answer themselves as if they are the dolls. Dolls that will 'do things', such as close their eyes or cry 'mama', help to create a relationship between children and dolls. The doll often becomes the friend of the child, the same as a teddy or other soft toy. I have written elsewhere about the important relationship between an infant and their first toy (*Creative Storytelling with Children at Risk*, 2004).

However, as with many other toys, modern dolls seem to do too much and leave little to the child's imagination. I have seen many children get increasingly frustrated when they struggle with dressing and undressing designer dolls that come with sets of clothes for every occasion. I recall my own frustration at wasting time crawling round the floor to find a tiny white plastic shoe at a children's party! If children are given the basics then everything else will be created through the imagination.

In puppet playing, the puppet takes on the character for the duration of the play and is a mouthpiece for the playwright or storyteller, or child or adult. It is important to remember:

Whereas a child or an adult will talk *to* dolls, they will talk *through* a puppet.

Children will also speak through various toy figures when telling a story and will create scenes with the family in the doll's house. A doll with moving limbs that can sit or stand or turn the head is almost a puppet. Dolls with articulated joints have been found in the graves of children in several countries. Early examples of grave dolls have been found in Peru and Egypt, where dolls made of rags or stone have been buried with the child. The British Museum has a Roman rag doll dating to 3,000 BC that was found in a child's grave.

Large wooden figures with moving limbs, known as *automata*, are still used in processions and celebrations of religious festivals. For example, in Sicily they have the drama of 'Mary of the Kiss' on Easter day morning.

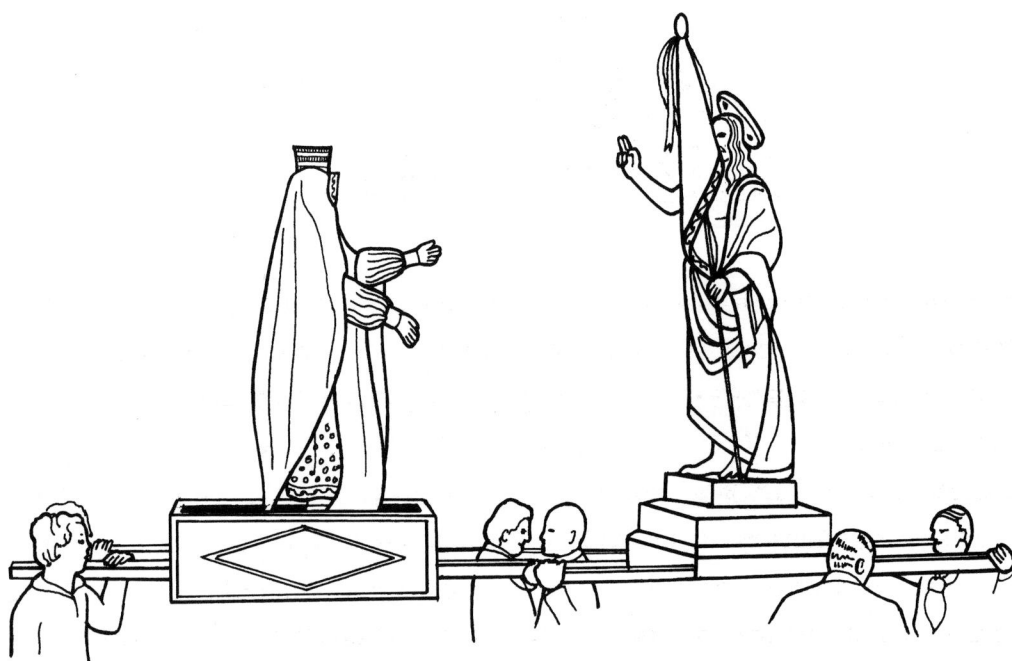

Large wooden figures of Jesus and Mary are paraded around different streets followed by crowds of hundreds. Eventually they see each other and Mary drops her black cloak of mourning and live doves fly up to the sky. The two figures move towards each other and when they meet, Mary embraces Jesus and kisses him. She blesses him and then blesses the crowd.

When I saw this celebration recently it took place alongside a true mixture of traditions. There were Gypsies selling balloons of all kinds and colours and a child let loose a spider-man balloon which followed the doves into the heavens. The lemon-seller in traditional costume was encouraging every woman 'whether married or single' to buy his lemons. The whole 'performance' was a coming together of the old and the new.

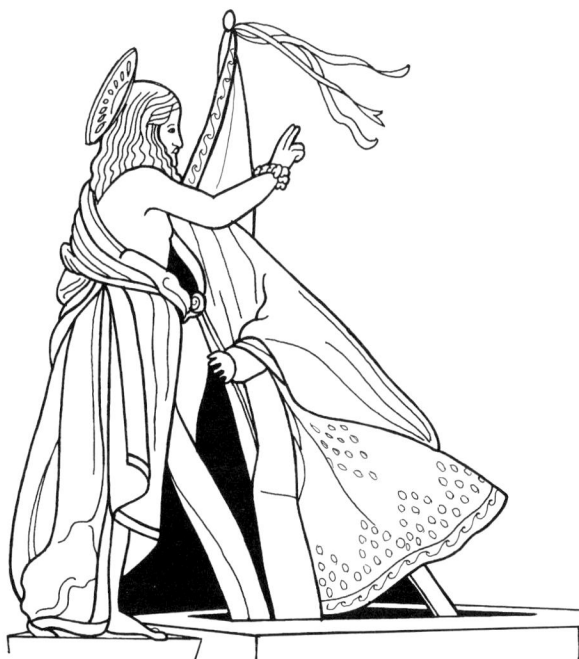

Shadow puppets feature in the ancient traditions of many societies including India, China, Indonesia, Malaysia, Turkey and Greece. Although many cultures had puppets as part of religious practice to tell sacred stories, this has changed over the years, and puppets are now used more for popular entertainment. Shadow puppets are thought to have developed from drawings and there is some similarity between the two-dimensional shape of the shadow puppet and the shapes of Middle Eastern and Asian art. (One can speculate, when did someone first make a shape with his or her hand that became a shadow on a wall?) Although some societies still use puppets to tell the ancient stories, many of these stories have been brought into the modern age and topical political themes and national figures are depicted through puppets. The use of shadow puppets, once a classical art form, is declining in most countries through the advent of television and cinema.

Shadow puppets are traditionally made from leather although nowadays they may be made of paper or card. When I was in Malaysia there was one shadow puppeteer who used to go into the hospital to have his chest X-rayed and would then steal the X-ray plate in order to create his puppets! One could occasionally see his vertebrae showing through the paint if one was able to inspect his puppets at close quarters. Although shadow puppets only appear as black silhouettes when they are held against the white screen, illuminated by a light bulb, they are in fact all painted in traditional colours according to their characters.

In ancient cultures, shadow theatre was associated with ritual dramas. In Greece, shadow theatre is still performed today; it has a long history of change and development that probably had its roots in ancient Turkey – more precisely, one should say the Ottoman culture that spread over the Balkans and Asia Minor. Historians disagree with the more ancient origins: some say that shadow theatre was influenced by Hindu Gipsies, others that it came from China through nomadic Turks.

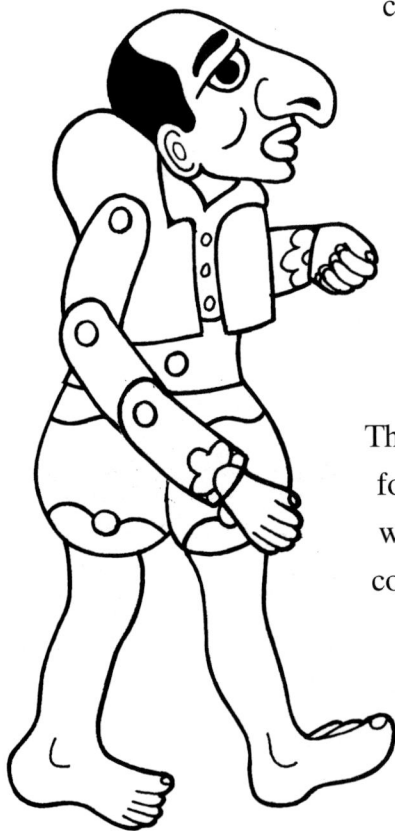

The main character Karaghiozis, is eponymous for the Greek shadow puppet theatre as a whole. There are three types of plays: popular comedies in which everyday life situations are enacted, plays that depict fairy tales and legends, and those stories that depict heroic themes, especially during times of wars and social upheaval.

Karaghiozis is the central comic character who represents the poor people struggling against oppression. He lives in a shack and gets involved in all sorts of situations, and usually ends up being beaten. He is portrayed with a long arm because he is always engaged in petty theft. He is a larger-than-life character who gets himself into all sorts of scrapes. There are other stock characters that are always represented by a recognisable shape and stance, and we shall meet some of these characters later in the book when we create our own shadow puppets and stories.

Many of the children and adults with whom we work will relate to these characters and will want to create ones of their own. The Magic Tree that usually stands in the centre of shadow puppet plays from most cultures is a very special 'anchor'. The tree creates a safe place and will transform any creature that abuses the space. The Magic Tree features in some of the stories that we tell in the following chapters.

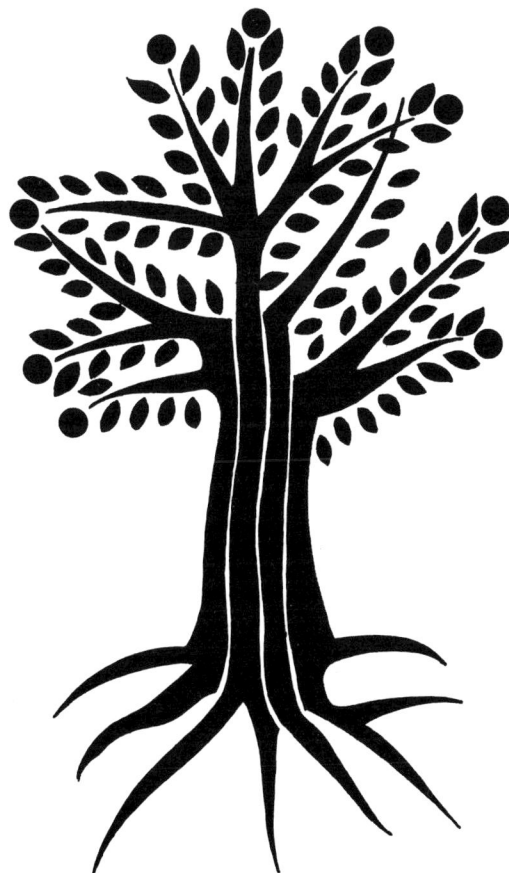

In Sicily there is a specific, hand-made wooden puppet that can move with metal rods (rather than the strings of marionettes). The puppets are used to tell the epic stories, (that are often sung in a special voice chant) from the days of the wars of Charlemagne. The tale, known as a *Chanson de Geste*, originated in France and spread to Italy and Sicily as well as England. The original manuscript is in the Bodleian Library in Oxford. Episodes can be taken from this extremely long text and adapted to puppet playing.

The troubadour tales usually depict four main characters: Roland, Oliver Angelica and the Saracen, and the tales are still performed in places like Palermo and Syracuse. *Stories of Roland Told to the Children* (Marshall, 1907) can be used as a resource for creating plays. The wooden puppet depicted below can be copied and painted on card or indeed created in wood or wire. Unless of course you are fortunate to have a holiday in Sicily where they are readily available for purchase.

The ancient art of puppetry was once as powerful and popular as other artistic traditions such as drama and music. Sadly, there are very few puppet theatres left in the UK and Europe, and in Asia puppet activities are also in decline. For many children, and indeed adults, their experience of puppets is limited to animated figures on television or robot figures with moving limbs in space stories.

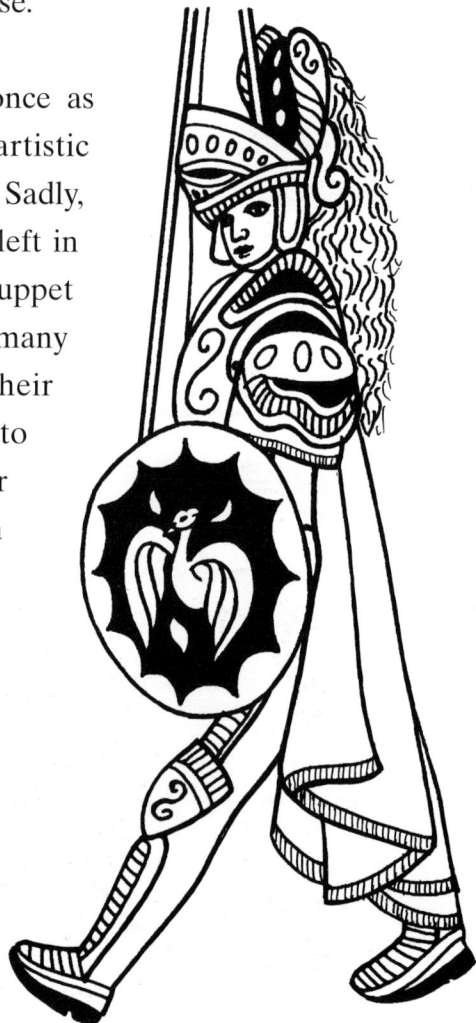

Sicilian Puppet Roland

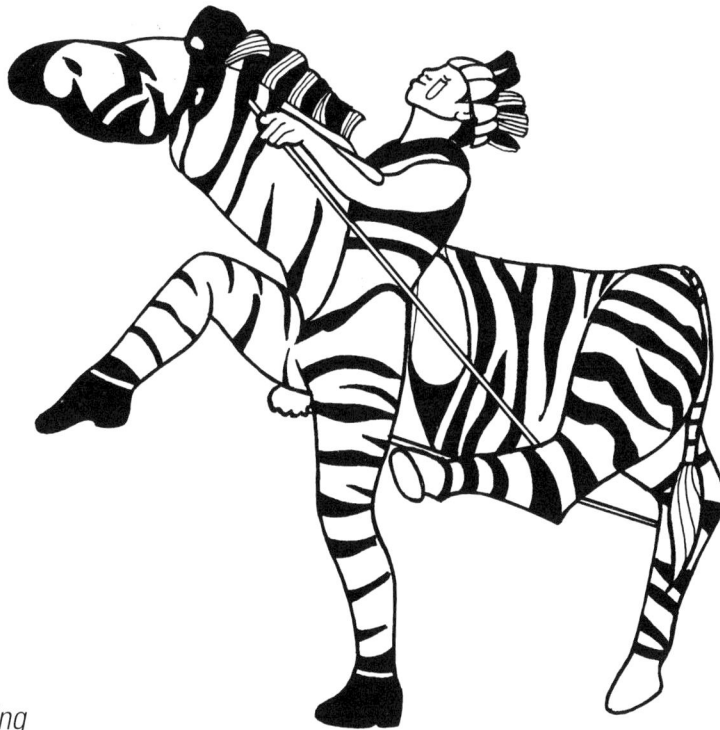

The Lion King

The art of puppetry is now left to a small number of dedicated followers. However, puppets seem to be making a come-back to our theatre as we can see both in The Royal Shakespeare Company's production of *Venus and Adonis* and in *The Lion King* in the West End of London. Both productions

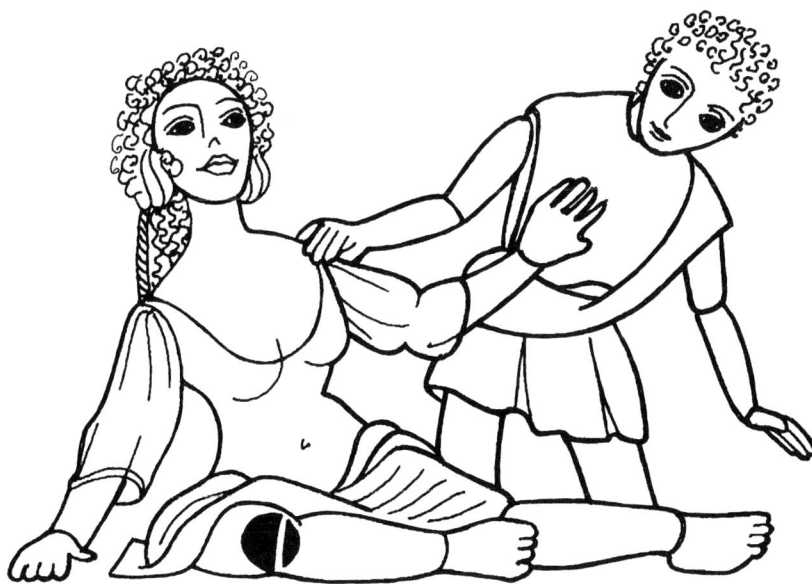

Venus and Adonis

have sumptuous life-size puppets, and the actors have had to learn new skills in order to manipulate them within the smooth running of the plays.

There are references to puppets in the plays of Shakespeare and Ben Johnson where puppets also form part of the bigger play. All of Shakespeare's references to puppets are derogatory. For example, comments such as:

> Fie! You counterfeit, you puppet, you!
> (Shakespeare, *A Midsummer Night's Dream*, iii.2.288)

and

> Thou, an Egyptian puppet, shall be shown in Rome ...
> (Shakespeare, *Anthony and Cleopatra*, v.2.208)

In Ben Jonson's play *Bartholomew Fair* people are referred to as puppets that can be manipulated, and there is also a puppet performance towards the end of the play. The puppets comment on the actors and in turn the actors comment on the Fair and the world outside – each being a metaphor for the other.

> BUSY: And my argument against you is that you are an abomination; for the male amongst you putteth on the apparel of the female, and the female of the male.
>
> PUPPET DIONYSIOS: *You lie, you lie, you lie abominably.*
>
> COKES: Good, by my troth; he has given him the lie thrice.
>
> PUPPET DIONYSIOS: *It is your old stale argument against the players, but it will not hold against the puppets; for we have neither male nor female amongst us, and*

> *that thou mayest see, if thou wilt, like a malicious*
> *purblind zeal as thou art!*
>
> (The puppet takes up his garment).
>
> LEATHERHEAD: Not that it enhances meaning but we will put it
>   in and gracious!
>
> *This tragical encounter falling out thus to busy us,*
> *It raises up the ghost of their friend Dionysus,*
> *Not like a monarch, but the master of a school,*
> *In a scrivener's furred gown, which shows he is*
>   *no fool.*
> (Ben Jonson, *Bartholomew Fair*, v.5.322–325)

Ben Jonson uses the device of a 'play within a play' where members of the audience interact with the puppets and the puppets improvise their responses. Within the puppet play and the improvisation people are speaking important 'truths' through the puppets. These truths may be philosophical or a commentary on the deeper meanings of life or indeed a metaphor that can be healing or challenging. These truths speak both to individuals and groups of people, young and old. It is an important function of puppet plays, that we utilise in education as well as in therapy.

CHAPTER 2

Fun with Fingers

IN THIS CHAPTER WE ARE LOOKING AT THE IMPORTANCE of the human body as a starting point for puppet work and the importance of the body being 'warmed up' and not tense. Special attention is paid to the hands and fingers. We use children's singing games for developing the imagination that leads into simple puppet work through drawing faces on fingers. We then describe how to make simple finger puppets from paper, fabric and old gloves. There are worksheets for making these simple finger puppets together with stories and exercises.

The human body is the most creative and flexible of communicating creatures. The body can run and jump, dance and sing, and create a myriad of shapes and patterns. Usually we use our hands and arms to express ourselves when we speak as well as the facial expressions produced by dozens of tiny muscles.

Sometimes a single finger is used to make a point, or both hands and arms to suggest that something is enormous. We might wave goodbye with a very small hand movement or give a gigantic wave through our whole arm if someone is in the distance. If we want to signal something very important then we would use both arms in a series of giant waves over the top of our heads.

Let us use these movements that I have just described, to warm up the body for puppet work. Indeed we can pretend our whole body is a puppet and move as if we are a marionette, a 'Puppet on a String'.

Warming up the Whole Body

Use a rhythmic piece of music to dance round the room making very big patterns. You can run and jump or make a series of leaps. Stand still and make the largest waves possible, as if someone is a long way away. Stand far enough away from others so you can stretch out both arms. Turn round in a circle first one way and then another. Walk round the room with legs and arms held very stiffly. Walk round again as if your arms and legs are made of jelly! Pretend that your intelligence is in your knees and find another pair of knees to have a conversation.

Warming up the Arms and Hands

Make small hand waves as if someone is just across the street. Shake your hands several times, and then stretch your fingers wide and close your hand tight in a fist. Look at the back of your hand and then the palm and notice its uniqueness. Measure your hand against someone else's hand and be aware of similarities and differences.

Circle the wrists outwards and then inwards. Hold your palms together and press them. Use the thumb of one hand to massage the palm of the other and then change over. Repeat the massage on the back of the hand. With the thumb and middle finger of one hand, massage the wrist of the other and then change over.

Fingers as Finger Puppets

Hold up one of your hands, make the fingers move individually and you have five finger-puppets. They can bend and stretch and they can dance; you can let them hide away by wrapping your thumb inside your fingers as you make a gentle fist or they can fly away like a flock of birds. Link your thumbs together and create a butterfly movement (see Worksheet 2.1 at the end of the chapter).

1 Stick a small label on the fingernail of both index fingers, curl the other fingers away and place both fingers on a flat surface in front of the child. Move your fingers alternately and say the following rhyme. As you say the fly away line, let the bird 'fly away' and bring your middle fingers back. Similarly on the last line let the index fingers come back.

Two little birdies sitting on a wall
One named Peter, one named Paul
Fly away Peter, fly away Paul
Come back Peter, come back Paul.

> **The advantage of this rhyme is that it does not involve touching the child. There are other rhymes where fingers act as puppets where touch is involved so care must be exercised. Please be aware of protocols for child protection and whether there is any history of abuse. In any case touch must be agreed not imposed.**

The following touch rhymes involve 'safe' body areas (hands, arms and toes) and encourage sensory development and body awareness. They each have a rhythm and a brief story structure (see also Jennings, in press, *Creative Play with Babies at Risk*).

2 Hold the child's hand and use two fingers to 'walk' round the palm during the first two lines, take two big steps up the arm on the third line, and gently tickle under the arm on the fourth line.

Round and round the garden
Walks a teddy bear
One step, two steps
Tickly under there.

3 'This Little Piggy went to Market' is another body rhyme, this time using the toes but it can be adapted to use with fingers. Start with the big toe and hold each toe for each line of the rhyme and on the last line run the fingers up the side of the leg as far as the knee (or up the side of the arm as far as the elbow).

This Little Piggy went to market
This Little Piggy stayed at home
This Little Piggy had plum pudding
This Little Piggy had none
And this Little Piggy went 'squeak, squeak, squeak' all the way home!

4 Incy Wincy can either be done up the child's arm with the appropriate movements or without touch, using both hands in front of the body. The child can also mimic the sound and movements.

Incy Wincy spider
Climbs up the water spout
Down comes the rain and
Washes poor Incy out.
Out comes the sun
And dries up all the rain
Incy Wincy spider
Climbs up the spout again.

Worksheet 2.2 at the end of this chapter describes how we can make spiders.

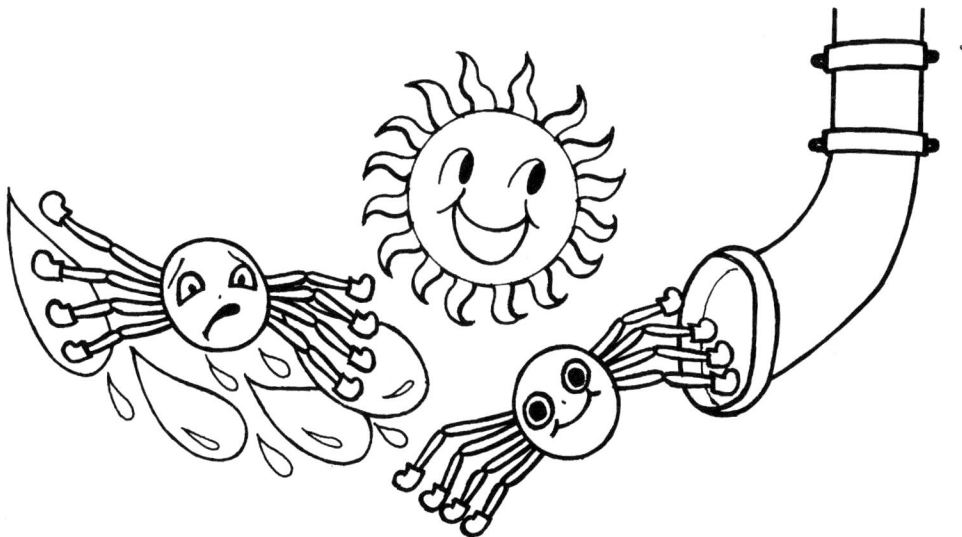

Finger Faces

With a water-based non-toxic pen, draw a face on a fingertip of each hand and let them have a conversation. Create a face on all the fingers of one hand and tell a story about these people or creatures as you move them. You can do this with a child as a way of introducing puppet work, or the child or children can create it for themselves. Do make sure that the colours are non-toxic and child (and parent!) friendly.

If you are working in groups then two people can allow their fingers to 'talk', but it is a good idea to suggest that the fingers do not touch, otherwise it could lead into a battle!

Simple Paper Finger Puppets

It is a good idea to practise this for yourself before doing it with the child or the class, but it is the simplest way of creating a finger puppet 'in the moment'. It does not have to be kept unless you wanted a display. However, the most important thing about puppets is that they are used in action and stories (like masks), rather than being hung on a wall.

Cut a small strip of paper (photocopying paper is fine) the length of your index finger between fingertip and the first joint. Stick the ends with sticky tape or paper glue so you have a small cylinder. Cut out a paper circle about 2cm in diameter and draw a face on it. Stick it with paper glue to the top of the cylinder and you have a simple paper finger puppet. The 'body' of the puppet can also be decorated. Some puppets have been coloured like Matrioshka dolls, or as members of a family or characters in a story. The important thing about this puppet is that it is easily accomplished which is especially important for low achiever children and for those who lack confidence in their own abilities.

Worksheet 2.3 at the end of this chapter illustrates all the stages for this finger puppet.

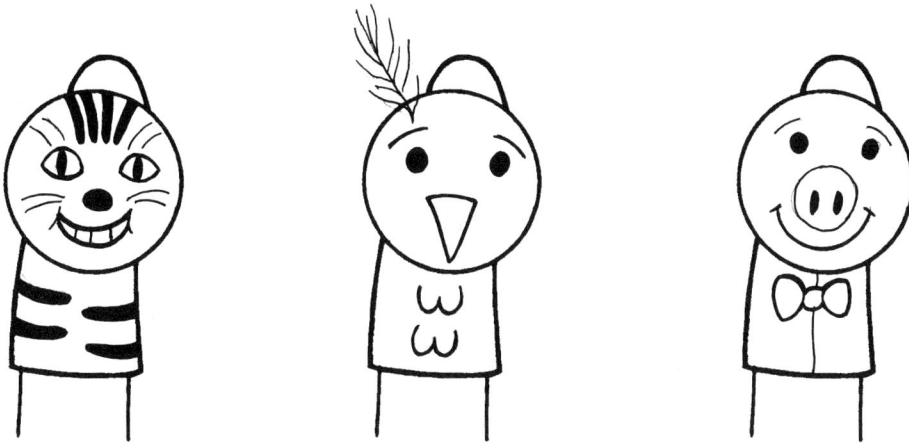

You can elaborate these puppets by adding a single item such as a feather or a sequin or a small button or some strands of wool for hair. There are other paper materials you can use such as the sections from egg cartons, pieces of lacy doilies, shiny paper, and the packaging from many cosmetics. You need to decide early on who is making the puppets. Younger children will find these small puppets very fiddly but you could prepare the cylinders in advance and cut out circles for small children. Older children can make their own puppet and really stretch their imaginations.

Fabric Finger Puppets

You can make your own finger puppets from a variety of materials, but felt is especially adaptable. The simple puppet is the same as with paper, and a felt face can be stuck on. For a puppet that is closed at the top you need to cut the material in two pieces and either stick or sew them along both sides and the top (see Worksheet 2.4). You may need to adapt the measurements for an individual child.

You can also make finger puppets by knitting them as small cones and then sewing or sticking them with decorations.

Easy-Peasy Finger Puppets

You can buy very cheap gloves from discount shops, or collect single gloves where one has been lost or search the jumble sales. You will soon have a collection of fabric and knitted gloves and will have no conscience about cutting off the fingers!

You will have plenty of 'fingers' to create a collection of puppets that you may make for yourself and have as part of your collection, or you might run a finger puppets project with an individual or a class.

If you have acquired the gloves, please make sure they have been washed or dry-cleaned. If they are knitted gloves, then you will need to catch the stitches to stop them unravelling – either sew or lightly glue them.

If you are creating your own collection then you can be really adventurous with buttons and sequins, feathers and ribbons, scraps of net and fur fabric, beads from broken necklaces and odd earrings. You can stick with white glue or sew or staple the additions to your finger puppet. Some people have embroidered or crocheted their puppets' faces and clothes. The creative possibilities are endless. Sometimes it is fun just to let the puppet character emerge without having a set plan, and you will soon find that it becomes an art form in its own right.

> **Please be aware of health and safety if you are working with small children and make sure that there are no parts that can be swallowed, especially if a child may choose to suck a puppet.**

If you are creating these finger puppets with small children, please remember that they are very fiddly and that can create frustration and loss of self-esteem. Keep the material very basic and use a glue stick rather than white glue as it is easier to handle and dries very quickly. Usually children over the age of seven years can manage these puppets unless they have coordination difficulties. You may want to start with the simple paper puppet described above before trying the material finger puppets.

Worksheet 2.5 gives the basic ideas for making these puppets, and games and stories for their use.

Reflections

Remember that the creating of a puppet, however simple, is not an end in itself. Puppets are not just artistic products. The creation of a puppet is a means to an end. The puppet is brought to life through actions and songs and stories, and then it truly lives!

Worksheet 2.1
Fingers as Puppets

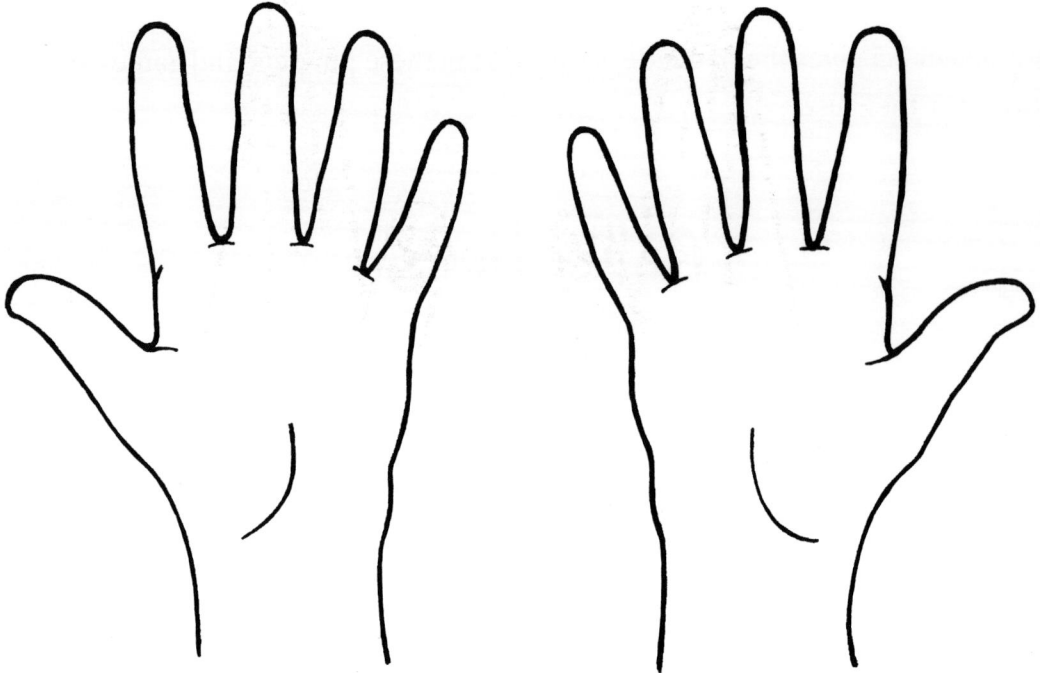

'let your fingers dance'

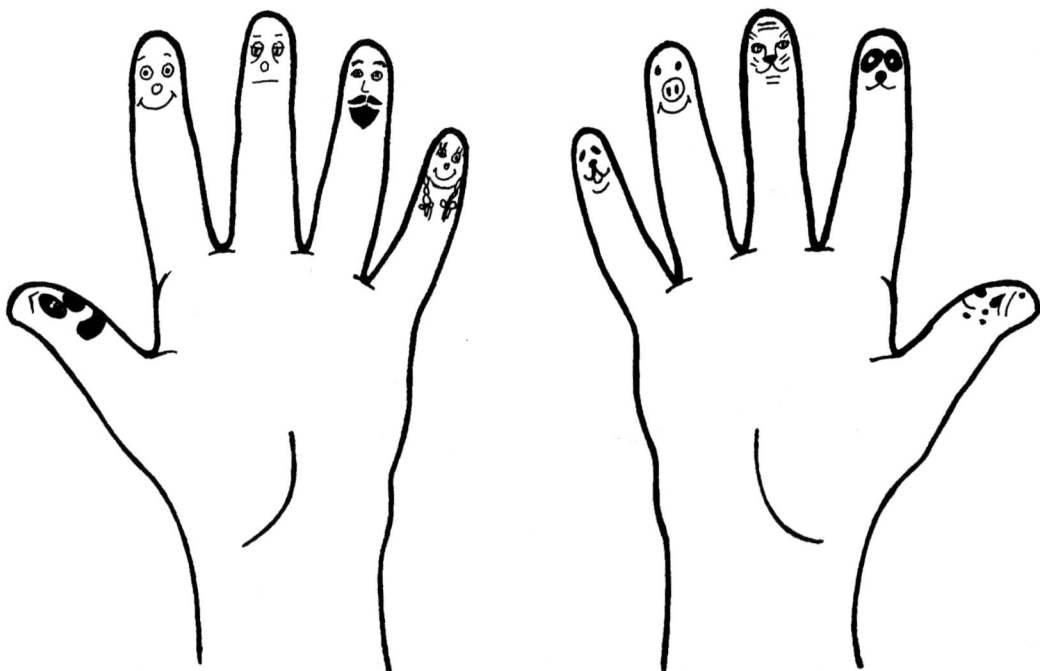

'all different people on your fingers'
fingers can dance and play and talk to each other

Worksheet 2.1
Fingers as Puppets

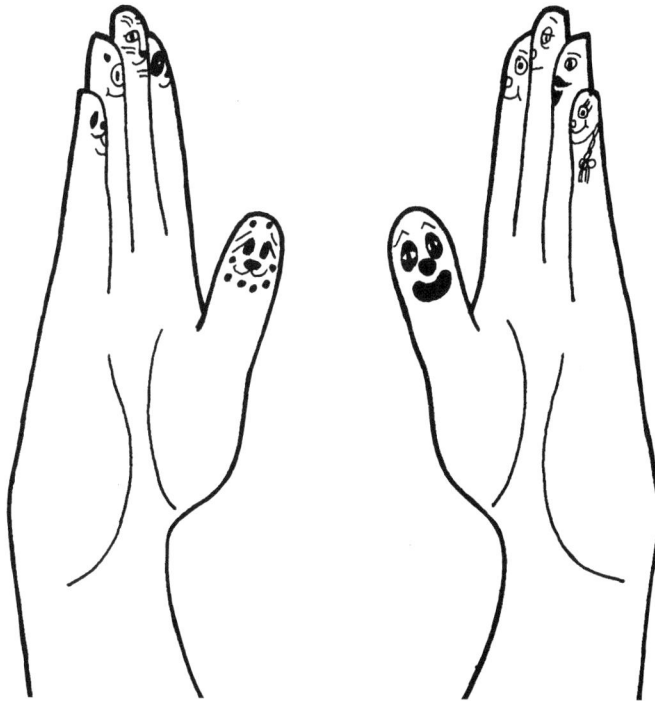

'having a conversation with other puppets'

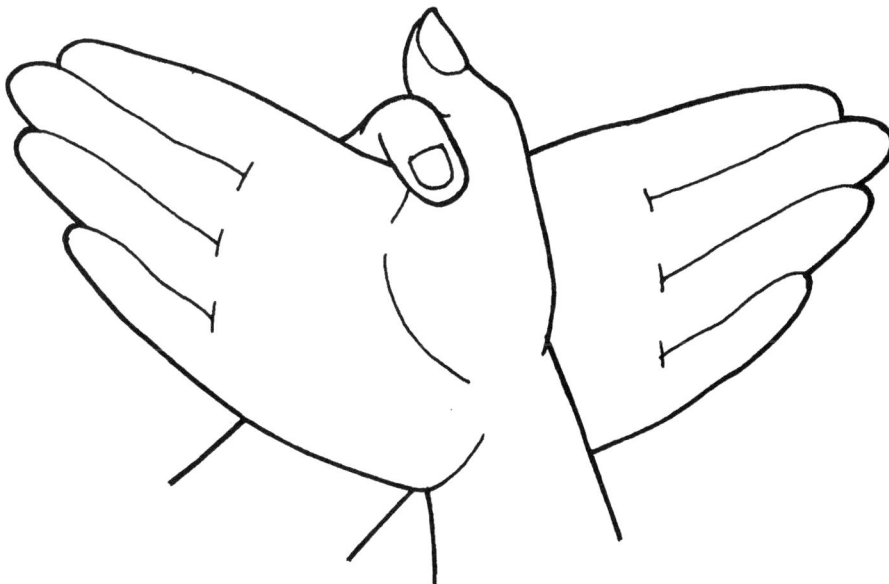

create a butterfly by linking thumbs and spreading your fingers; maybe you can all let your butterflies fly round the room

Speechmark

Worksheet 2.2
Spider Puppets

Side 1

To make a basic spider you will need five pipe cleaners and some coloured thread or wool.

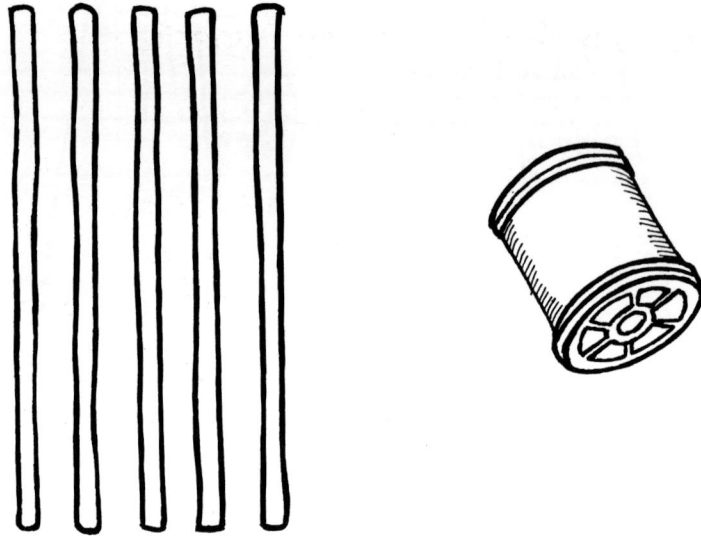

Take four pipe cleaners and twist them round several times in the middle. Use the fifth pipe cleaner to create the head and the body and bend round the centre of the four.

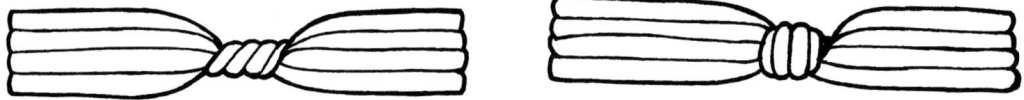

Separate out the 'legs' and bend them in the middle so that your spider can stand:

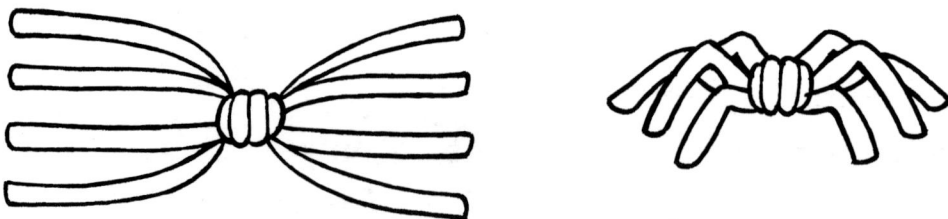

You can use thread or wool to make your spider whatever colour you want: wind it round the limbs and body. Leave one long thread so you can hold your spider.

Worksheet 2.2
Spider Puppets

Playing with Spiders

Hold your spider up by its string and make it bounce up and down. It can meet other spiders. You can move the spider as you say the Incy Wincy Spider rhyme:

Incy Wincy spider
Climbs up the water spout
Down comes the rain and
Washes poor Incy out.
Out comes the sun
And dries up all the rain
Incy Wincy spider
Climbs up the spout again.

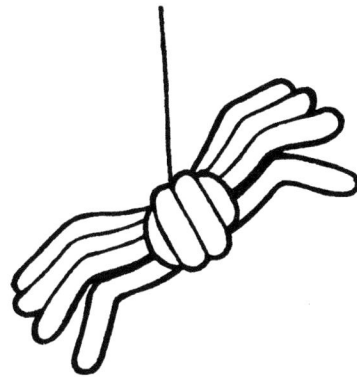

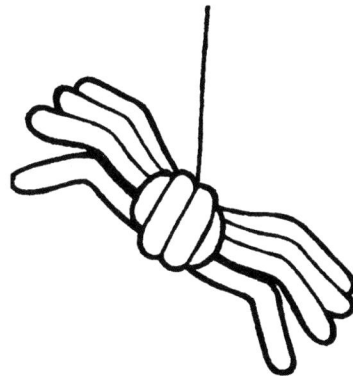

To turn your spider into a finger puppet, use another pipe cleaner to create a loop under the spider and you can insert your finger and make it walk!

Grandmother Spider

In native American tradition, Grandmother Spider is very wise and she created the very first alphabet so that people could write to each other. Grandmother Spider sits in the centre of all the 'dreamcatchers' so that she can protect children from their nightmares.

Worksheet 2.3
Simple Finger Puppets

You will need: plain paper, (100 g/m²), scissors, glue stick, sticky tape, coloured pens.

1 Cut strips of paper the length of the top of your finger to the first finger joint and wide enough to go round your finger plus a bit to overlap. Stick the ends to make a cylinder.

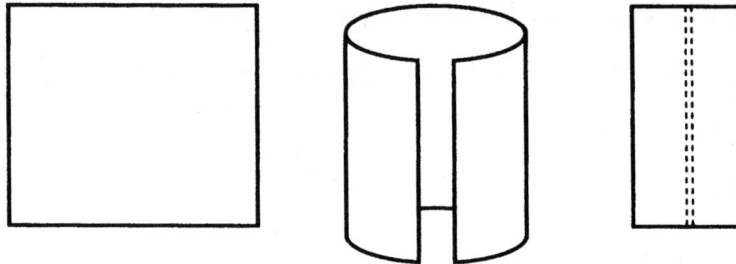

2 Cut circles of paper with a diameter of 2.5 cm. Stick the circle to the top of the cylinder with a dab of glue.

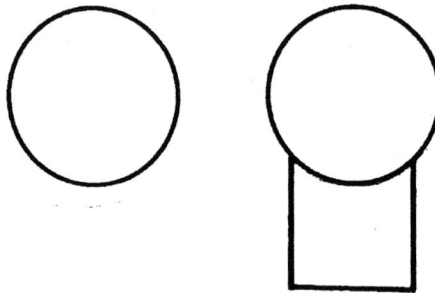

Now that you see how it fits together, you can repeat the exercise, but this time colour the body and create the face before you do the sticking. You can stick a few pieces of wool on to make hair or decorate with a feather or sequin.

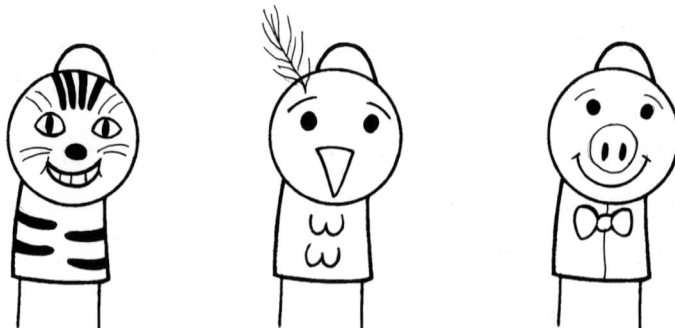

Worksheet 2.3
Simple Finger Puppets

Side 2

> Remember to create a comfortable space between the children and yourself when using a puppet – there is nothing worse than for you or them to feel that it is 'in your face'.

For Groups
- Create the finger puppets of the characters of a story that everyone knows and then tell the story.
- Let everyone create individual characters and let them meet each other.
- Make up a new story with a partner and then share it with others.
- Suggest to the group that they can make a group story with everyone's characters included.
- If there are issues around social learning, such as health and safety, bullying, diet and food, puppets can be created to explore and teach.
- The puppets can be used as ways into expression of feelings and emotional literacy.
- They can also be used in cognitive-behavioural learning for appropriate social skills.
- Some of the above techniques can also be used in one-to-one puppet work.

For Individuals
- The finger puppet may become the first means of communication for the child – and the character they create may have significance.
- The puppet can communicate things that cannot be expressed in other ways.
- The child may communicate through their finger puppet to your finger puppet.

Worksheet 2.4
Fabric Finger Puppets

You will need: pieces of felt (scraps from other projects are usually big enough), sharp scissors, glue stick, needles and coloured threads, feathers and other decorations (or coloured pens).

Cut two pieces of felt that will fit over your finger to the second finger joint and allow enough room for sewing them together.

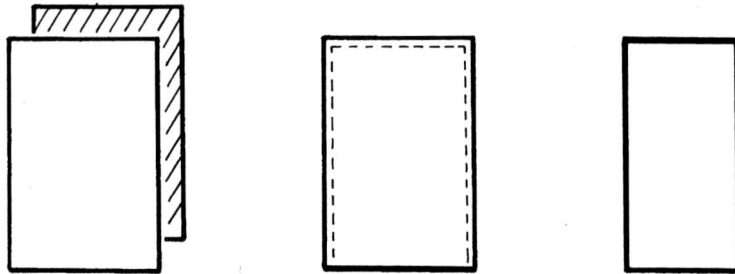

Sew them together either with overstitch along the edges or with a running stitch around both sides and one end. Make sure the puppet can fit comfortably over your first finger.

Your puppet is now ready for decorating, either by drawing a face with coloured pens or by sticking or sewing on pieces of felt, feathers or sequins for example. You may decide to cut out a face and stick it on with glue.

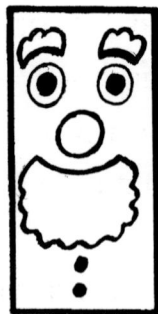

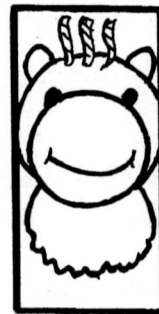

Worksheet 2.4
Fabric Finger Puppets

Variations and Stories

In addition to the materials listed you will need: pipe cleaners, scraps of other material, wool or embroidery thread.

The fabric puppets can become more elaborate if you so wish. For example, you can sew or stick on wool for hair, glue small pieces of pipe cleaner for arms, make a hat or a scarf or a bonnet. The possibilities are endless!

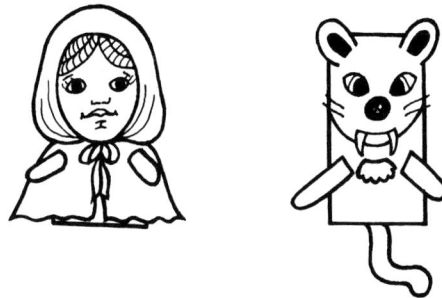

When working with children or adults using the fabric puppets, it is a good idea to make the simple paper one first, since this is a 'fail-safe' puppet. It also introduces the idea of the finger puppet that can then be elaborated. Because the fabric puppets are more painstaking, it is perhaps a good idea to focus on just one if you are creating them with other people. They can choose their own character, or the group can agree a story or myth they would like to tell.

Little Red Riding Hood is an ideal story to create with children (and many adults seem to like it as well!) or the Odysseus story where he is on the raft, tied to the mast, and the sailors with wax in their ears so they cannot hear, are rowing as hard as they can and the sirens are trying to tempt Odysseus into the water with their singing where he will surely drown.

The group themselves will also come up with their own ideas for stories.

Worksheet 2.5
Easy-Peasy Puppets

Side 1

You will need: assorted odd gloves (either of fabric or knitted), glue stick, sharp scissors, needles and thread, embroidery thread, sequins, buttons, wool, fur or fabric for decorations.

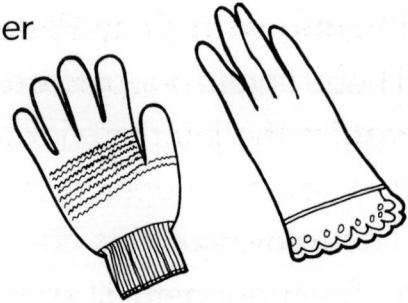

1 Cut the fingers off the gloves, making sure you leave enough length in the finger. You can always trim it again later if it is too long. If the gloves are knitted then catch the stitches round the base or glue them so it does not unravel.

2 You now have the base for your finger puppet that can be developed in a simple or elaborate way. One suggestion is to make it simple at the beginning otherwise it can become awkward and cumbersome and then bits drop off and there is general frustration.

3 Try gluing on eyes nose and mouth with sequins, buttons or fabric scraps.

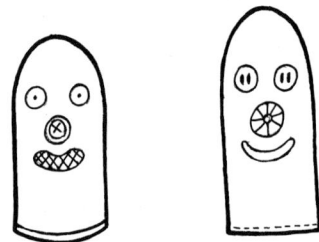

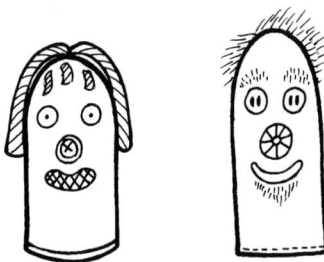

4 Now add some hair using wool, or fur fabric that can also be glued.

5 Now you can add simple clothes: a hat or scarf, a skirt or trousers – all by cutting out material and sticking it on.

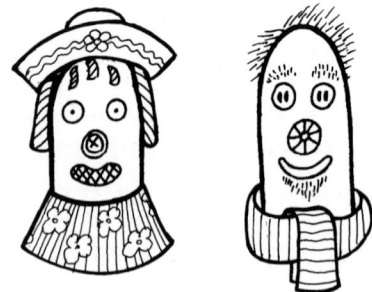

You can do the whole of this exercise by sewing everything instead of gluing. You can also sew the features on the face.

Worksheet 2.5
Easy-Peasy Puppets

Playing with Easy-Peasys

These finger puppets are fun to play with because they do not restrict the joints and the material moves easily and flexibly.

- Allow the puppets to move around and find their own way of moving.
- Each puppet will start to develop its own style.
- What voice does your character have?
- The puppet will start to have its own personality.
- Let your puppet interact with the other puppets.
- Create a scene between two or three puppets and show to the group.
- Imagine the puppets are taking part in a debate or a business meeting. How would they communicate?
- Pretend the puppets are members of the school council. What are they talking about?
- All the puppets came from the same glove – imagine they are members of the same family. How will they relate to each other?
- Suppose all the puppets are marooned on an island. Who would take on the different roles? How many leaders are there?
- Ask the group to suggest different situations where the puppets can interact.
- Invite the group to choose a story to enact through the puppets.
- Perhaps they would prefer to make up their own story?

Easy-peasys can be used with individuals as well as groups and can be a part of therapy or creative activities. As they all come from the same glove, there are interesting themes to explore about 'attachment' and relationships.

CHAPTER 3

Simple Dolls and Puppets

THIS CHAPTER WILL FOCUS ON VERY SIMPLE INTERVENTIONS with puppets and dolls and offer ideas on how they can be used to develop basic activities for emotional literacy, and individual personal stories.

We will look at the most simple of dolls and puppets that children can make or that we can make ourselves for working with the children. These are all puppets and dolls that will give the greatest scope for the children's imagination as well as being vehicles for education, therapy and pleasurable play. They also have the advantage of being low cost and replaceable if necessary. I am indebted to Gayle Kearney for the idea of the cotton hand and finger puppets that she uses in her play therapy work.

I have chosen the easiest fabrics for us to work with, as for adults and children alike, things that are 'fiddly' just increase our frustration. I took ages to be able to cope with making small things and surpassed myself when making a dress for a Story Doll – instead of cutting an opening for the head, I cut through both sides of the dress! My ingenuity had to find braid to sew on to cover up the extra slit!

It may be that we do decide to purchase ready-made puppets for our work but it is important to remember that many of them are not washable or mendable. Puppets that have been dribbled on, dragged around the floor or generally mutilated may make us think twice about the best equipment for our meagre budgets.

Of course we have the ground rules and contracts with all of our groups and individuals but they are not infallible. Children with severe disabilities may well dribble without control. Children with behavioural difficulties will often test the rules and massacre a puppet with glue and paint or pull its head off. However, it is equally important that the children are allowed to use equipment and that toys are not locked away. If we overprotect things they may never get used. I have seen a play room where the toys are kept on a high shelf: 'The children will only break them' said the staff! This was on a ward for children with profound disabilities, where there were no activities and the children rocked and moaned. They had never been allowed to play so no wonder the toys were broken.

We can also overdo the hygiene rules. Obviously we need to be aware of health and safety issues and make sure that with all the materials that we comply with EU or any country's health and safety standards. However, the following example must act as a cautionary tale.

I was working in a nursery for children with mixed and multiple disabilities and the students from the local art college had designed and created a special mattress for stimulating through texture and sound. The children were able to explore the different fabrics such as corduroy and satin, simulated fur and hessian. If they pressed in certain areas there were squeaks or rings or growls. It was a great success until the nursing staff said that they were covering it all with plastic so that it could be washed down. The upshot was that the children lost all interest in the mattress!

Obviously we will take care with small chewable parts that can be swallowed, or stuck up noses or into ears. But this needs to be balanced with an awareness that children also need to learn about taking risks. If they are overprotected then they will never learn about what is dangerous and what is safe, what is kept outside the body and what can be taken inside. Furthermore, we know that an over-clean environment is likely to increase a child's susceptibility to infections and can contribute to allergies and a lowering of the immune system.

Puppets and dolls, like masks, are to be *used* rather than hung on walls or kept on shelves. They are an extension of ourselves and enable the telling of stories and the playing of plays.

Choosing between Dolls, Puppets and Masks

In the scheme of things dolls, puppets and masks are in a developmental progression, as described in the following bullet points:

Dolls

- Dolls are usually talked *to* by the child and maybe asked questions.
- The child can 'role-reverse' and answer them self 'as if' they are the doll (as we get older, we do this in our heads).
- The exception to this is the use of 'feeling dolls' described below and Story Dolls described in Chapter 9.

Puppets

- Puppets are objects that the child talks *through* to someone else: a teacher, a friend, an audience, a therapist.
- Puppets move their limbs and sometimes their features.
- Puppets may also talk to each other: the child having a puppet on each hand or two people each having puppets.

Masks

- Masks are like puppets that we wear – instead of talking through the puppet – we take on the character of the mask.
- Differences between masks and puppets reduce when we have paper plate puppets that we can hold close to our faces.
- The broomstick puppets (see Chapter 5) are almost masks, as we hold them in front of ourselves.

Cotton Finger and Hand Puppets

The Flexible Friend

This cotton finger and hand puppet is probably the simplest and most flexible (see Worksheet 3.1).

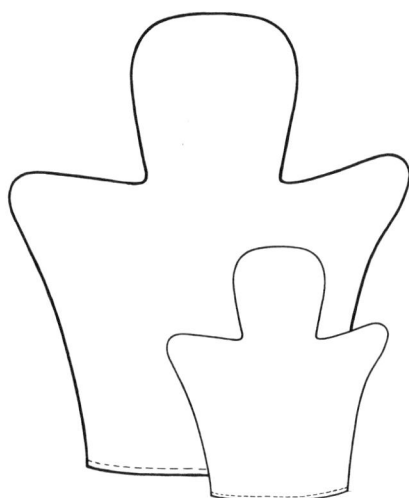

It can be coloured with crayons or coloured pens:

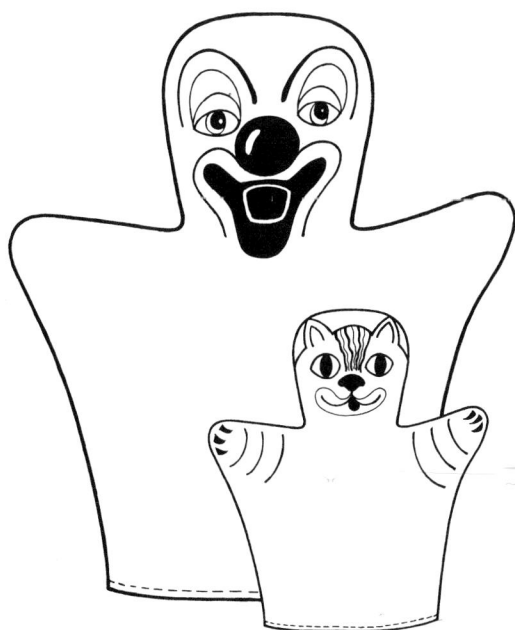

Or you can make it more elaborate by sewing on hair or sticking on features:

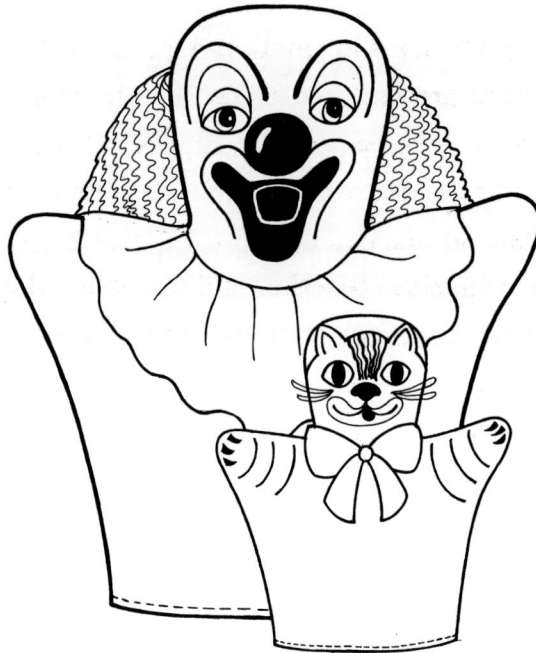

However, the most important aspect of this type of puppet is its very simplicity and the fact that it is fail-safe. Any child can create a face, even if it is three dots. Some children may not even want to create a face if they are feeling invisible or lacking in confidence. The blank face may tell you exactly how they are feeling and a therapeutic story may be about how the character 'found' a face.

How to Use the Puppets

Therapeutic Play

If you want to work with free choices and non-directively, have several of these puppets and drawing materials and follow the child's actions. You can reflect back to the child what they are doing without guiding or leading them. They may ask you to be a part of the story. Check out who they want you to be or what they want you to do, without assuming anything. The more you can follow the child without interruption or imposition, the more the child will tell the story that they need you to hear.

Emotional Literacy

These puppets can also be used in emotional literacy with children under the age of ten years. There are children whose emotions are so confused that they need to get back to basics. The puppets can be used to represent different feelings and the child can be invited to draw an angry face, a sad face, a happy face, and so on. You may want to warm-up to this exercise by looking at books or magazines together and discussing the different feelings that people are expressing. You can use the worksheets on feelings in *Creative Play with Children at Risk* (Jennings, 2005), pages 64–67. There are also feeling stories in this book that can be adapted for puppet work such as 'The Children of Lir' and 'Red Riding Hood'.

It is also important for the development of emotional literacy that children are able to differentiate degrees of feeling. What is the difference between feeling cross and feeling angry and feeling furious? Many young people are unable to experience a spectrum of feeling and explode with volcanic rage at a seemingly small incident. By drawing the feeling face on the puppet, the child can then express the feeling, name it, look at what triggers it and why. Then explore possible changes and practise them.

Creating a Feelings Puppet

The Seven Stages

Stage 1

The child draws a very angry face on the puppet.

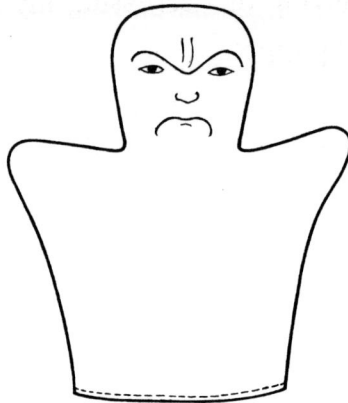

Stage 2

The child is encouraged to express the feeling – perhaps in relation to another puppet – through sounds or words.

Stage 3

The child is encouraged to name the feeling. Is the puppet: Cross? Angry? Gutted? (You can make a list of as many angry words as possible and the child can tick whichever is appropriate for them.)

Stage 4

What triggers that feeling? For example: Being ignored? Losing?

Stage 5

Do we know why this feeling is triggered?

'No-one has ever listened', 'I have to win' or 'I'm a dodo'.

Stage 6

Clarify whether the situation can change, for example by discussing whether it possible to be noticed or heard (by changing my behaviour?) or do I have to accept the situation and therefore practise decreasing my feelings slowly?

Stage 7

Depending on the answer to the previous question, I can use role-play to practise new ways of behaving or decreasing my extreme feelings. I can create a 'before' and 'after' puppet.

You can close this exercise by drawing and colouring the appropriate feeling on another puppet, eg, irritated rather than angry. See if the child can identify the feeling for themselves.

You can design your own seven stages using the above as a model for your planning. For instance you might want to assist a child to move forward from being very shy or withdrawn so that their feelings are more accessible and expressible. Ways to help can be discussed in Stage 6. If you are working with mourning and loss a child can be helped to express their feelings through these puppets in varying degrees of intensity.

The puppets can be used with small children in groups for an emotional education programme, where feelings are linked to situations. We feel … when we are … Be sure to have discussions with the children about their ideas and check that your ideas are relevant with cross-cultural groups. There is no universal expression of emotion, it is context and culture specific.

Creating Feelings Dolls

The Feelings Dolls work on the basic emotions, and enable the expression of feelings in an appropriate way. These dolls are simple enough for children to make and then identify the feelings expressed by the doll.

This doll is made from felt material and is cut out in two pieces. The basic shape is shown here; there is a to-scale pattern on Worksheet 3.2 at the end of this chapter.

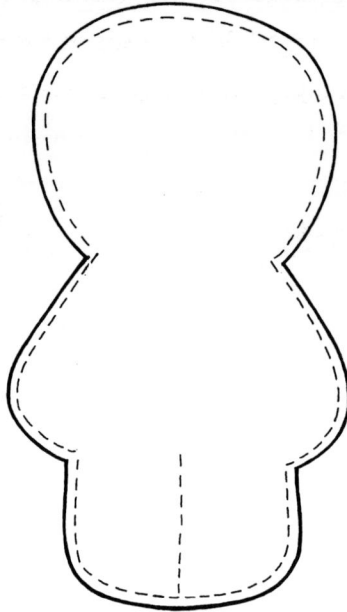

This is the basic doll that can then be dressed and given hair:

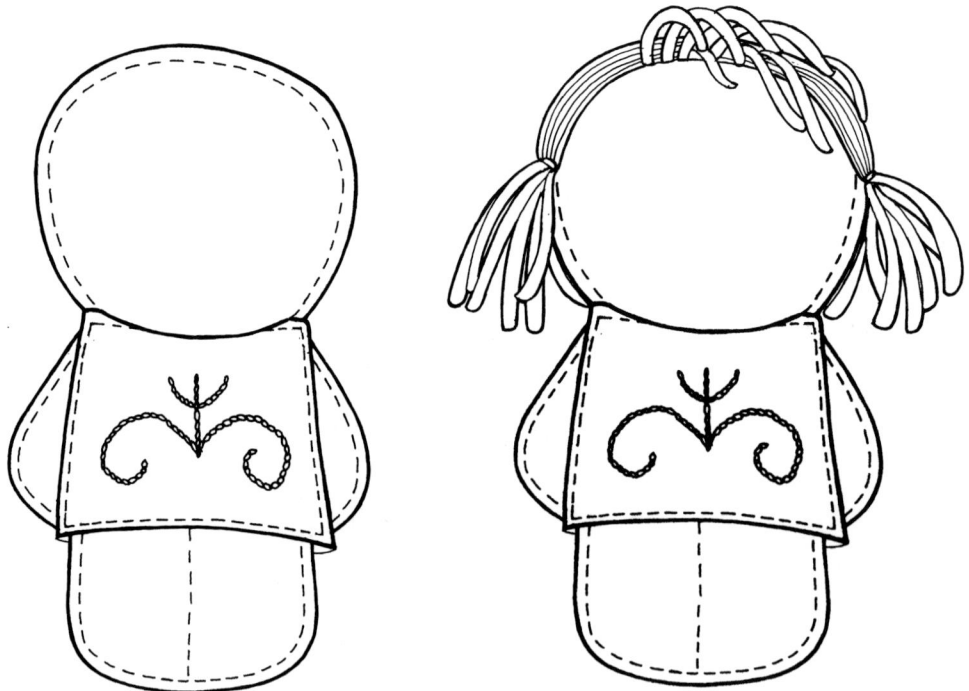

You now have a two-sided doll and can indicate different feelings on each side. For example, the one that I have shows the doll with a smile (made with chain stitch), and two embroidered eyes on one side. On the other side are closed eyes and a down-turning mouth (embroidered with chain stitch). One side is happy; on the other side, is it sad? Angry? Most adults say it is sad when I ask them, but some children think it is 'sulking', 'in a strop', 'switching off', 'crying', 'angry'.

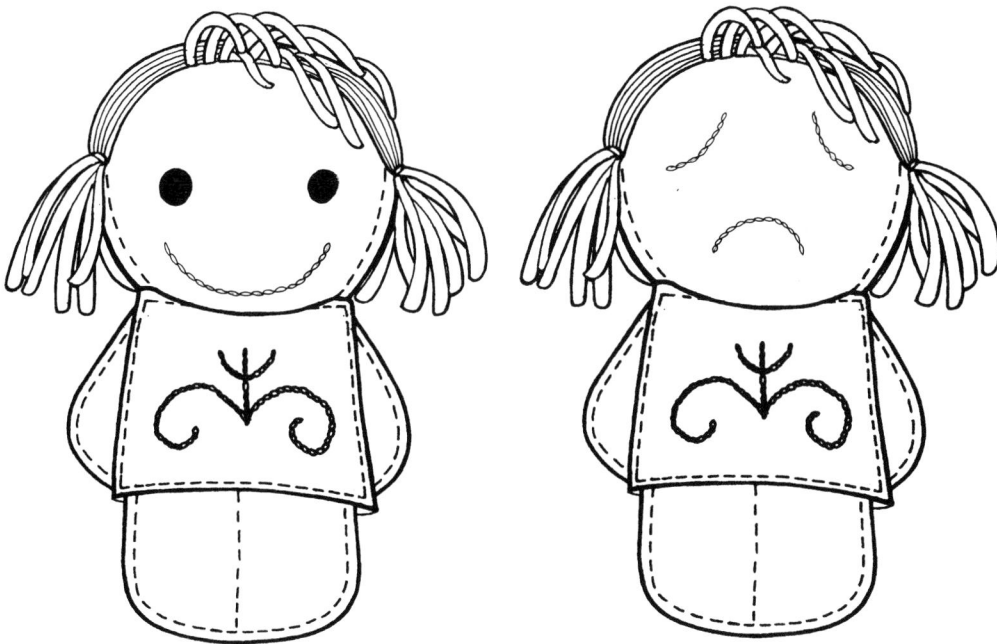

This doll can be used to explore feelings for developing emotional literacy as well as for expressing outside and inside emotions. For example: the face that the world sees and how I really feel; my face when I am with other children and my face when I am on my own.

Some children immediately think of the rhyme:

> There was a little girl
> Who had a little curl
> Right in the middle of her forehead.
> When she was good
> She was very, very good but
> When she was bad she was horrid.

Storymaking

In Chapter 9 there are many ideas for creating Story Dolls based on the elements and great mythic figures. These dolls can also be a means of creating new stories for children who need to express changes in their lives. For example, children who felt happy when they lived in one house (or attended one school) and then felt sad when they moved to another house (or changed school). Conversely, a child who has been abused may first show the sad/angry face of the doll and then the happy face now that they are with a safe family.

> **The simple Story Doll is a reminder that sometimes adults can get too complicated and sophisticated about children's lives and their feelings. Sometimes we need to acknowledge very simple stories and simple expressions.**

Simple Story Doll

This simple doll shape can be created the same sizes as the pattern on Worksheet 3.3: large or as a miniature doll, a 'Pocket Venus'. You can create another size by just changing the size on the photocopier. The doll is in the shape of Venus, a gentle goddess of love who was venerated by the Romans who adorned her with roses, (it was centuries later that she became associated with sexual love). She loves order in her garden, especially strawberries and herbs, and her jewel is the emerald.

Her links with herbs make her an ideal figure to develop sensory work by collecting and differentiating fresh herbs. Telling stories about gardens, and planting seeds, (see *Creative Play with Children at Risk*, Jennings, 2005) are activities that are especially helpful with children whose lives are chaotic. Being able get 'back to basics' in the environment and in nature are very soothing experiences and they can help to create stability.

Creating a Simple Story Doll

The basic doll shape shown below is the simplest Story Doll that you can make, but it will assist you in all sorts of directions in stories and activities. Usually you can make it in felt but it can also be made in other materials that have a firm, close weave.

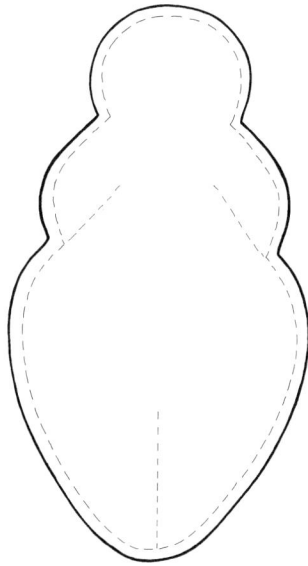

The advantage of this doll is that the nipples and pubes can be indicated with small flowers without offending anyone's sensibilities:

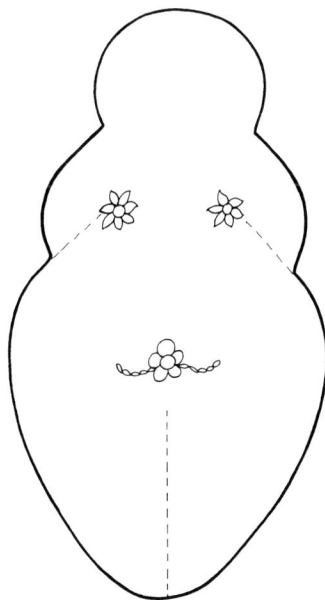

However, these do not need to be represented and if you prefer not, just sew the facial features and navel.

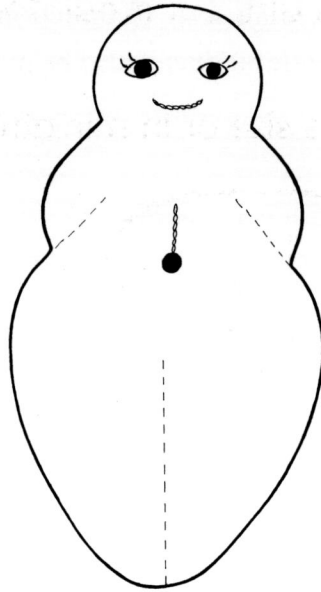

Worksheet 3.1
Cotton Glove Puppet

Side 1

This is the basic pattern for the glove puppet. Use a firm, close-weave cotton and cut it out double.

You can make it this size or in miniature for a finger puppet.

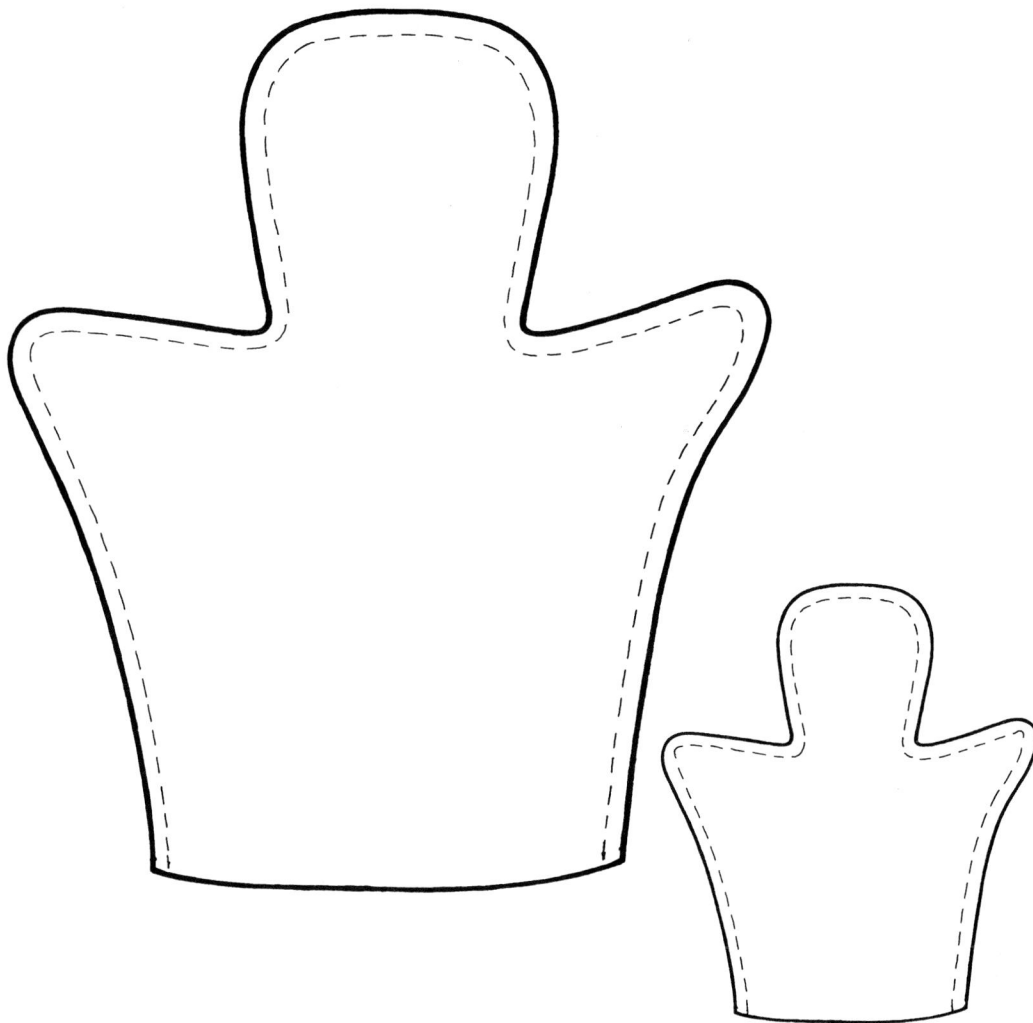

Machine or back stitch the pieces together along the stitch line. Turn it inside out and you have your puppet.

You can add hair using wool, and sew features if you want to establish the puppet's identity. Otherwise leave it blank for the child to colour or stick things on.

Worksheet 3.1
Cotton Glove Puppet

Side 2

Here are some children's ideas for different faces and expressions on these puppets.

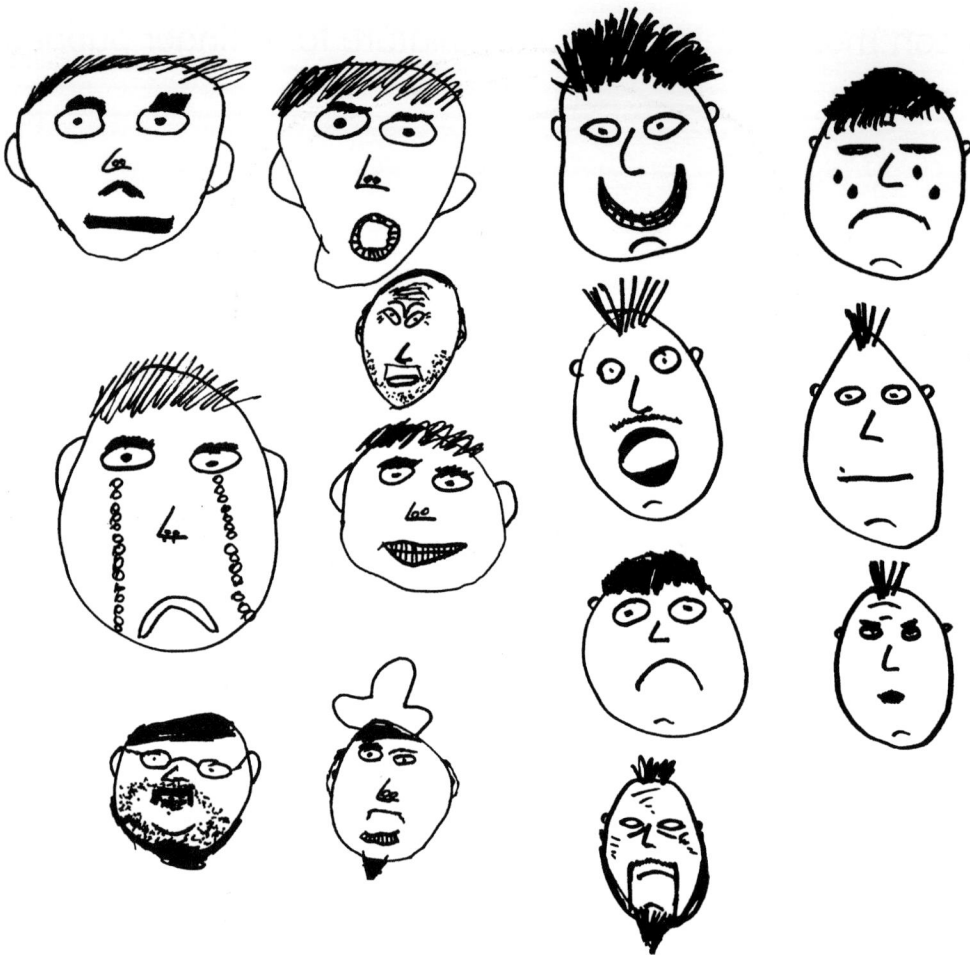

Use the puppets to explore feelings and stories as for the two-sided Feelings Doll on pages 40–41 in the text.

Worksheet 3.2
Feelings Doll

Side 1

Pattern for the two-sided Feelings Doll as described on pages 40–41 in the text.

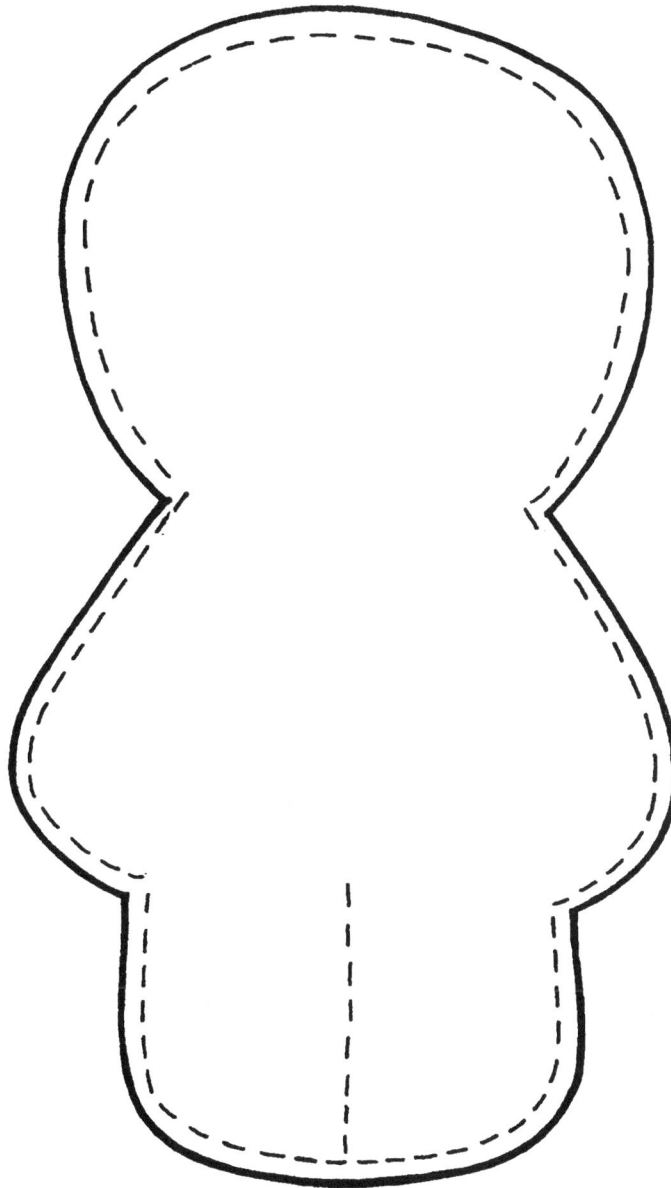

Machine or blanket stitch round the edges, leaving a small space for stuffing and then sew up. Follow the stitch line for the legs and arms.

48

Worksheet 3.2
Feelings Doll

Side 2Side 2

Cut out the dress, possibly a different colour for each side, and stitch across the neck and side as indicated on the doll according to the pattern.

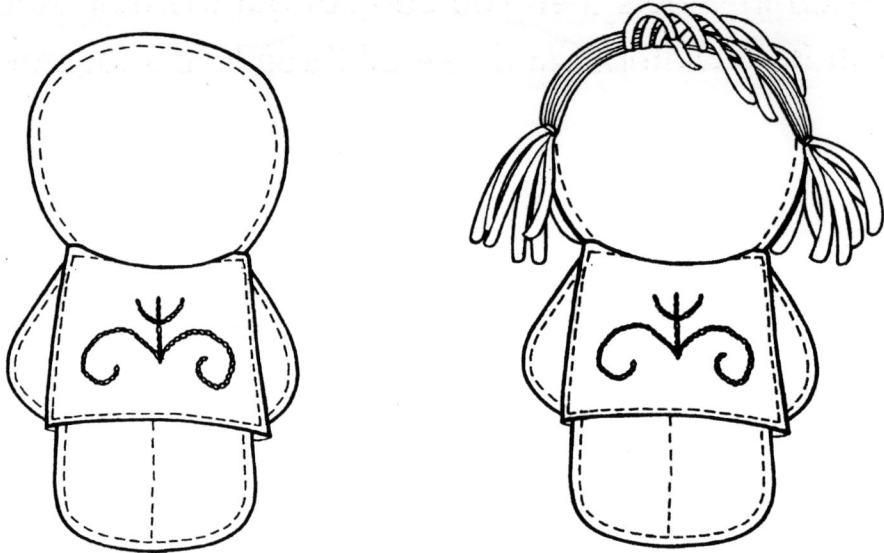

Choose a hair colour and use wool to create hair across the top of the head, ending in bunches on either side; sew it in place on each side and the top. Take shortened strands to create a fringe back and front across the top of the doll. Sew facial expressions on each side of the doll.

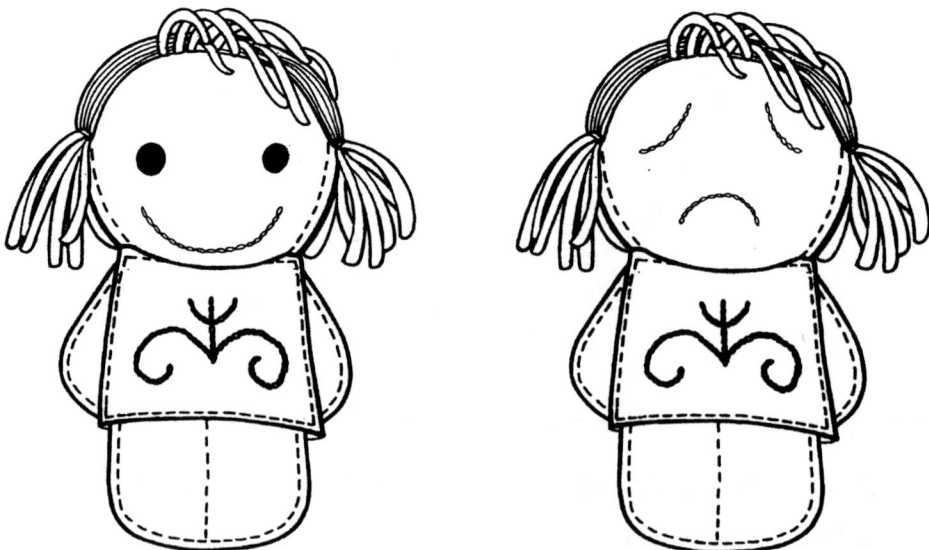

Worksheet 3.3
Simple Story Doll

Side 1

This basic doll is made from felt in two pieces and then sewn or stuck together, leaving a small hole for the stuffing before finally closing it up. If your stuffing is supplied in sheets then you can cut out the doll shape in the stuffing material and sew all three layers together.

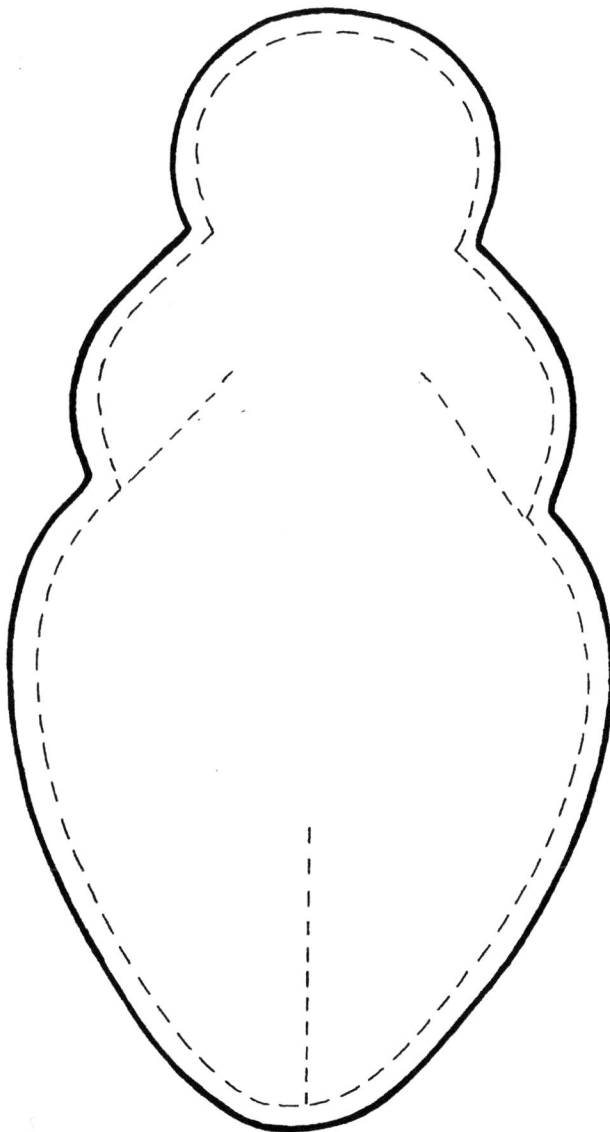

Hand sew with backstitch, or machine a line that goes through all layers to indicate the legs and sew a curve on each side to represent the arms.

Speechmark

P

Worksheet 3.3
Simple Story Doll

You can now embroider the flowers on nipples and pubes or the facial features and navel. You can add hair if you wish.

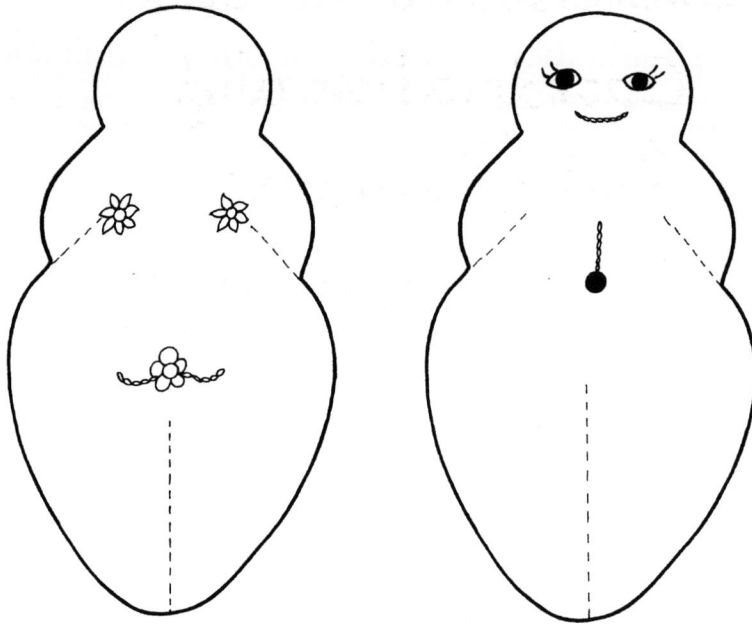

If you wish to create the Pocket Venus then use the following template:

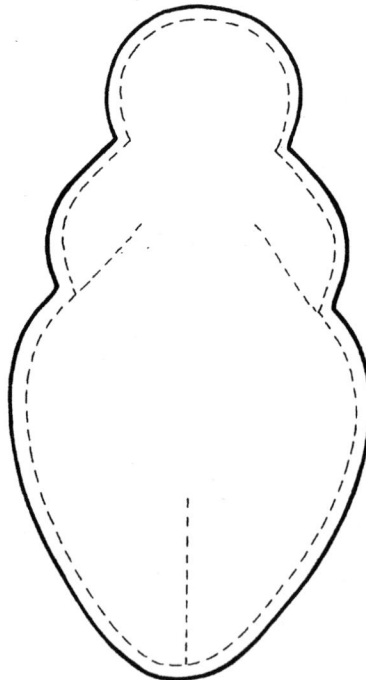

CHAPTER 4

Hands as Puppets

Exercises to Increase Coordination and Body Awareness

THE WARM-UPS FOR FINGER PUPPETS described in Chapter 2 are also useful introductions to working with hand puppets. We can add the following developments and extra exercises. Vary the techniques so that you and your groups or individuals do not become bored. The whole idea is to increase body awareness and coordination, and then to focus on the hands as a medium for expression.

1 Use some light hand cream or body lotion and massage your hands very thoroughly. Examine your hands closely and look at their unique qualities: the delicate tracing on the palms, the pattern of veins, and the shape of your nails. Remember just how individual your hands are: your fingerprints are different from everyone else's unless you are an identical twin.

2 Stand or sit with your feet firmly on the floor. Gently rotate your shoulders alternately: six times on one side and then repeat on the other. First rotate them inwards and then outwards. Try rotating both shoulders at the same time both inwards and then outwards. Each time do the exercise six times. Shrug your shoulders without making sudden movements, and then see if your shoulders can touch your ears!

3 Focus on your elbows: look at them one way and then turn your arms and look at them another. Put your hands on your shoulders and let your elbows 'talk' to each other. Cross your arms over and put your hands on opposite shoulders; give yourself a hug!

4 Put on some rhythmic music – whatever takes your fancy – and start moving your hands and arms: make them dance. Try to feel your hands coming alive and that they can tell all the stories that you want. Move your arms in big shapes as you are telling a big, big tale; move them in really small patterns as you describe something in minute detail; move your hands high as you tell a really tall tale! Your body can tell stories without saying one word.

Communication Using Hands

Observe the way that people use their hands when they talk to each other. Think about the variations among people from different cultures: some people talk with a lot of hand gestures, others with only a few. Notice how public speakers use their hands to make a point about something: fingers can point or beckon, both hands can welcome, a finger upraised can underline something that is being said.

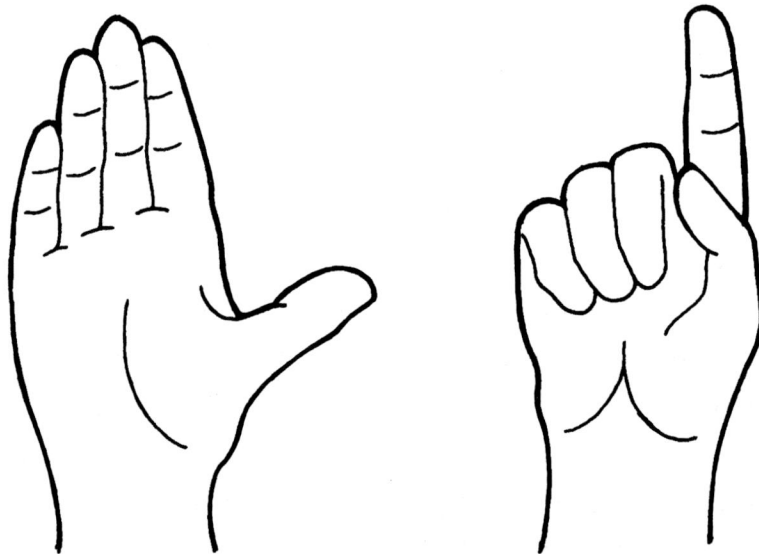

Think about all the 'languages' that only use the hands. Most people will now be familiar with TV programmes that are signed and there are several alphabets for communicating with our hands. Copy some of the signs that are used with a partner and see whether you can understand each other. The Internet has many pictorial systems that you can download and learn from.

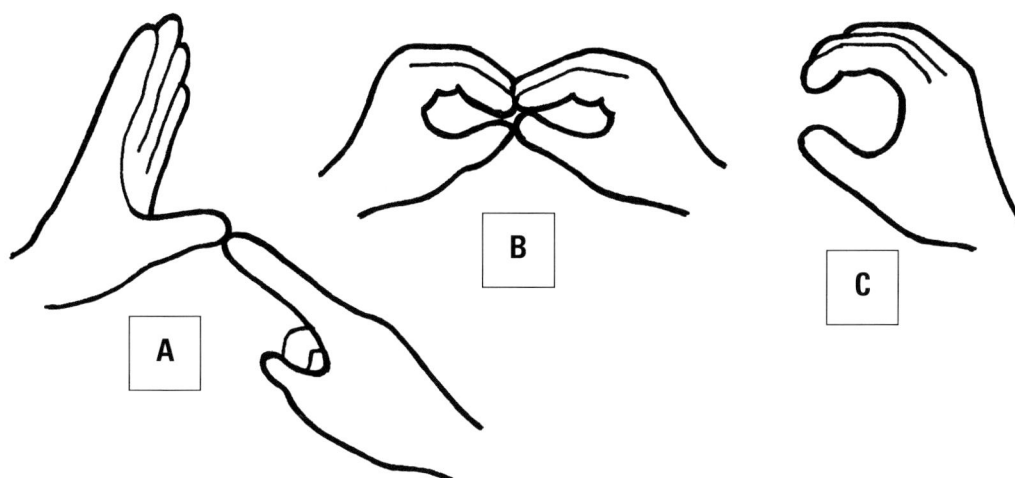

The following address gives you all the different sign systems: <http://www.deafblind.com/ukthma/html>. There are differences between the British Sign Language (BSL), the American Sign Language (ASL) and of course those languages that have different alphabets, such as Greek and Russian.

There are also more complex 'gesture systems' that can tell whole stories. For example classical ballet has its own set of gestures that involves the hands, arms, the face and sometimes the whole body. In the ballet *Swan Lake*, the swan princess describes how this lake (she gestures to the lake) came from my (gestures to herself) mother's (crosses her hands over her chest) tears (uses both hands to indicate tears flowing down her cheeks). In India there are several gesture systems through which it is possible to tell whole epic stories from their ancient tales. These are just brief examples of how our hands can be communicative. They can express feelings and atmospheres or can be very specific and spell out whole words.

Remember that one of the most devastating punishments in existence is for a person to have their hands cut off. For many people it would stop them being able to care for themselves, even to feed themselves, and it would completely change their capacity to communicate.

The story of Sedna from the Inuit peoples tells a very moving tale of Sedna who had her fingers chopped off by her father, and what happened to her and her life. Sedna can be made into a puppet or into a Story Doll (see Chapter 3).

The Transformation of Sedna (an Inuit Story)

Sedna is a beautiful young woman who is thinking that it is time to leave home and marry and settle down. None of the young men who come to visit her pleases her until one day she spies a handsome stranger in the distance. She agrees to go to his home and he removes his cloak and puts it round her shoulders. He then changes into the stormy petrel bird and flies with her to his nest on the cliff tops. The nest is very dirty and Sedna wishes that she had never come, and she sends a message out through the air and hopes that her father can hear it.

Her father does hear her and takes his kayak and paddles to where she is waiting nervously, as the petrel is only out of the house for a short time. She clambers down into the boat and her father starts to paddle. The bird sees them and dives down closely because he loves Sedna very much. There is a storm blowing up and her father becomes scared and wishes he had never come. He pushes her out of the boat hoping it will appease both the bird and the storm. Sedna hangs on with her fingers clasped around the edge of the boat but her father will have none of it. He takes out his axe and with a swift blow he cuts off her fingers. Sedna holds on again with her other hand and her father hits again and then again. Three times and all her fingers have gone to the bottom of the sea and turned into sea creatures.

Sedna herself floats to the seabed and she gradually turns into a mermaid or silkie and befriends all the creatures under the sea that love her dearly. She looks after the land and all the animals and the hunters have to ask her permission to hunt. If they break the traditional rules of hunting Sedna will send terrible storms and the local shaman has to visit her to intercede.

The shaman has to cross through difficulties such as a cauldron and a fierce dog before he can meet with her. His first task is to comb all the seaweed out of her hair because she has no hands. Then and only then will she listen to his request.

Sedna in the end forgave her father for the terrible deed of chopping off all her fingers but she stayed with the sea-life that had befriended her. She continues to punish hunters who do not care for the environment and she tells stories to the sea creatures that had befriended her.

Activities that Focus on Using Hands

The following exercises will help you to be more aware of the possibilities of hand puppets and there will be more variations when we look at shadow puppets in Chapter 6. The simplest shadow puppet is, after all, the shadow of a hand on a wall.

Talking Hands

Let the fingers and thumb of one hand become a puppet that 'talks' to you or to another person; let both hands talk to each other. Try this exercise non-verbally to encourage the hands to be expressive. You can then develop it, first with sounds and then with words.

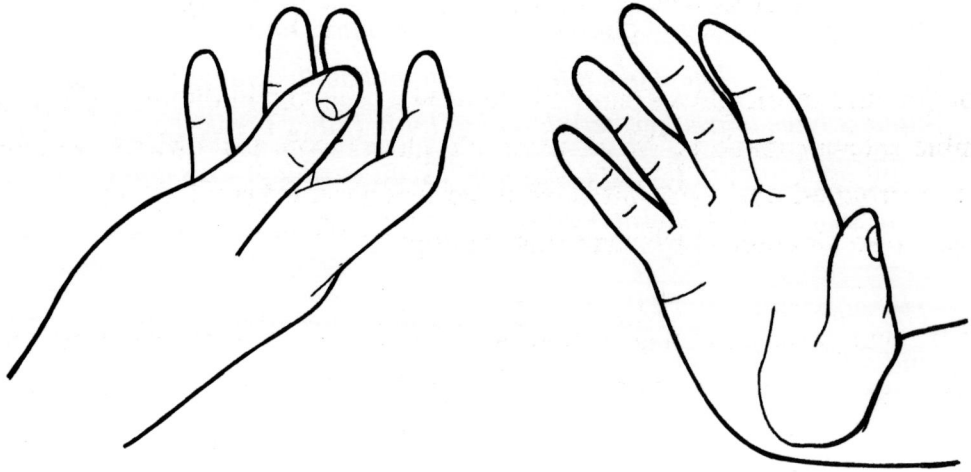

Fun with Hand Prints

- Mix some thick finger-paint (child-friendly paint with flour, or water-based cream or last year's suntan lotion).
- Create a picture with your own hand prints or create a group collage with everyone's hand prints.
- Use hand prints to create an individual or group tree with roots and branches.
- Hand prints can be used to make other kinds of pictures: portraits of others, landscapes, ourselves, animal heads, shadows.
- With clay or modelling dough (plain flour, vegetable oil, handful of salt and mix to a thick consistency), make use of all your hand muscles to make shapes and patterns.
- Make your hand print and measure it alongside everyone else's prints; can you see your own palm lines and veins in the print?
- When it is dry, paint your clay or pastry hand.
- Draw round your hand on stiff card and create a face or a family with paint or coloured pens.
- Make a collage with all the hands of the group.
- Build a three-dimensional model with all the hands of the group.
- You can stick a 'hinge' of card on the back of your painted hand of card and turn it into a puppet.

Making Glove Puppets

Woollen and fabric gloves can be bought very cheaply in discount shops or jumble sales or markets. We all have odd gloves from pairs where we have lost or dropped one. You may have fingerless gloves if you have cut off the fingers (see Chapter 2) to make finger puppets!

Put on one glove and imagine that it is a monster with tentacles or a giant spider. Let it 'slither and scuttle, creep and crawl, weave and writhe'. Use these expressive words to suggest and stimulate different movements, as they are very evocative. You can role model as the facilitator, demonstrating different ways of saying the words and then encourage participants to do the same.

You can elaborate the gloves by sewing on beads or sequins or lengths of wool. You can embroider eyes and nose and mouth. You can stick on felt cut-outs to make the face. Encourage the participants to create their own designs. They may even want to sketch their ideas for their 'creature' before trying to make it with materials and fabrics.

- Remember that you need to stick or sew on very lightweight materials, otherwise they will drag the whole puppet down and distort its shape.

- If you want a distorted puppet, use any materials to pull the glove out of shape. You can also stuff the glove with tissue paper or scraps, but leave room for your fingers!

As people get more confident with their glove puppet, you can improvise stories and plays. The puppets can react to each other in pairs and then in small groups. You can develop stories out of the characters that are created, and the group can have a storytelling workshop to make up their own stories. You can of course, start the other way round! If you or the group want to enact a particular story, you can then create the puppets to fit the story (see Worksheet 4.1).

Games and Stories for Spiders

See Worksheet 4.1 on how to create spider puppets from gloves.

1 Improvise with all the spider puppets and let them move together and separately.

2 Use an existing rhyme such as 'Little Miss Muffet' or 'Incy, Wincy Spider' to encourage playfulness.

3 *Grandmother Spider noticed that many of the children of the tribe were looking very tired. They felt sleepy during the day and could not concentrate. The elders and the parents became worried and asked Grandmother Spider if she had any advice. 'Encourage the children to talk about their dreams', she said, 'just in casual conversation when you are having your breakfast, and then come and see me again.' The parents did just that and were very surprised when their children told them terrible horror stories that even frightened the parents. They went back and told Grandmother Spider these terrible tales. 'Hm, I thought so,' she said. 'Well leave it with me and come back again tomorrow. But above all do not laugh at the children.' She started weaving webs as she thought and thought, and she had an inspiration. 'I will make the Dreamcatcher,' she said, 'and then I can devour the nightmares and bad dreams so that the children may sleep peacefully.' So Grandmother Spider gave every child a Dreamcatcher so they sleep peacefully at night.*

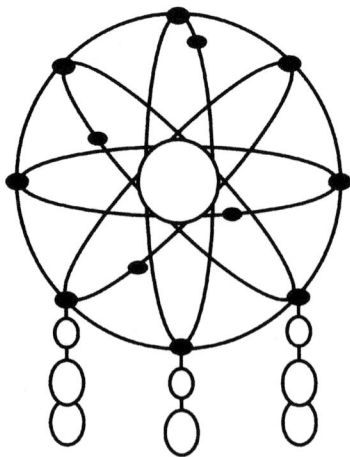

See *Creative Storytelling with Children at Risk* (Jennings, 2004) which has more about Dreamcatchers and Grandmother Spider.

Glove Puppets using Socks

All children will put socks on their hands and feet and pretend to be a monster or an alien. They will also spontaneously put a sock on their hand and pretend it is a puppet. Initially you can have fun with the socks and also use some of the warm up exercises described in Chapter 2 (see pages 14–15).

You can always find odd socks, or as with the gloves, find very cheap pairs of socks in all sizes and colours. Plain colours are best for making a more elaborate puppet with sewing and sticking. Coloured or stripy socks already give ideas for puppet characters, and socks with lace frills round the top lend themselves to making ballerinas or fairies.

The simple sock puppet works without making a mouth. You just sew or stick on the features, and any other additions that are needed. Buttons make round eyes, strong string can make a tail, fur fabric or felt can make ears, cut out paper or card can make teeth (see Worksheet 4.2).

A more elaborate sock puppet can have a moving mouth (see Worksheet 4.3) but has the advantage of not cutting the socks and losing stitches! Worksheet 4.4 gives some ideas about creating stories for sock puppets that you have made.

The Story of the Golden Stag

You can make sock puppets for the following characters (they can be the simple ones or the more elaborate ones):

Characters
Old man, old woman, young boy, young girl, stag's head, prince.

Follow the instructions in the worksheets and adapt to the different characters: for example, a hat for the old man, grey hair for the old woman, antlers for the stag, a crown for the prince.

Scenery

Paint the following pictures to create the scenery for the story. The pictures will set the atmosphere and the puppets can move from place to place.

- A poor house made of mud and sticks.
- A forest with lots of trees: everyone can paint one tree and cut them out to make a forest or paint one picture with many trees.
- One large special tree: you can get ideas from Chapter 1 (page 9).
- A palace with lots of turrets and windows.
- Flowers and garlands.

Many years ago an old man lived with an old woman and his two children. The stepmother hated the children and would starve and beat them, and everyone in the village knew that she was nasty and cruel. She said to their father that he must take them to the forest and kill them and although he pleaded for her to change her mind, she insisted. The children had been playing in the ashes and were covered from head to foot and as they followed their father into the forest, they left a white trail.

The father had not the heart to kill his children so slipped away while they were playing. The children called and called but their father did not answer, so they followed the white ashes all the way home. They climbed on the roof and kept warm where the smoke came through the mud and waited until they could hear their father.

The stepmother was furious that the children were home again and threw bones on the table for them to eat. She insisted that their father took them to the forest the next day, and this time they could not find their way home.

They walked and walked and the boy got more and more thirsty and went to drink rainwater from the tracks of a fox. His sister said, 'You must not drink that water or you will turn into a fox.' The boy was desperate, but he obeyed his sister. Then they found the tracks of a bear and the boy tried to drink the rainwater. 'No! No!', said his sister, 'You will turn into a bear.' They went on their way again, and came to the footprints of a stag, and the boy fell to his knees and gulped the rainwater. He turned into a magnificent stag and knelt in front of his sister and wept.

'Climb into the hammock of silver threads that is between my antlers, and I will take care of you,' he said. So she climbed up and swayed gently as he walked through the forest. He found a large tree and built a little house for her way above the ground. Each night he returned and brought fresh leaves and roots for her to eat and clear water for her to drink.

The prince was out hunting in the forest and was following the handsome stag that was returning to his sister. The prince saw that the stag was talking to someone, the most beautiful girl he had ever seen, and he knew that he wanted this girl to come to the palace.

He returned to the palace and called for his wise woman and said that she must find a way to entice the girl away from the forest and bring her to the palace. The old woman waited until the stag had gone looking for roots and went to the clearing in the forest where the tree was growing.

How do you think the old woman persuaded the girl to come out of the tree?

The girl went to the palace, and the prince was delighted to see her and said she would live like a princess until she decided if she would like to marry him. Meanwhile the stepmother heard about the new girl at the palace and came to check it out, because she herself wanted to marry the prince. She was able to turn herself into a young woman to entrap the prince. She followed the girl into the forest as she was picking flowers and gave her a potion to drink when she got thirsty. The girl went into a deep sleep and the old woman stole her clothes and arrived at the palace looking like the young girl.

The stag meanwhile was desperate to find his sister and searched high and low. Then he came to the palace and heard the prince calling his sister's name, 'Emily, Emily.' The stepmother rushed forward to the prince and the stag started to snort and paw the ground. The stag knew it was not Emily, and he recalled how the stepmother looked.. The prince was confused as to who was who! The stepmother said to him, 'Why don't you have your hunter's kill this stag – he seems dangerous.'

How did the stag escape being killed by the hunters?

The hunters found Emily in the forest and she was in a deep sleep. The prince fetched the wise woman to bring her out of her slumber. Emily told the prince the whole story and showed him how affectionate the stag was towards her. Meanwhile, the wicked stepmother was driven out of the palace and the prince and Emily had a beautiful wedding, accompanied by brother stag.

The three of them lived happily, and one day their father also came to live in the palace. He really regretted all that he had done and was pleased that the stepmother had never returned home.

So you have a story, the scenery and the puppets – have a great play!

The Pied Piper of Hamelin

You can use lots of rat puppets and let the other characters be played by the group or you can create all the puppets for the story.

Characters

You will need (as well as the rats): the Mayor, the Pied Piper, some children and some townspeople. Perhaps the children and townspeople could be finger puppets. You will also need a child who is lame.

Scenery

- Make a cut-out of the town hall and square for the first part of the story.
- Make a cut-out of a hill with a cave in the side for the second part of the story. You can then use the town hall again for the ending.

The town of Hamelin was plagued by rats and they were everywhere: in the houses, in the beds, in the kitchens. There was every different type of rat: black, brown, grey and white. There were even piebald rats. One day a stranger visited the town and said to the Mayor that he could remove the rats – for a fee. 'Anything, anything,' said the Mayor. 'Please remove them, they are driving us out of our homes, and of course we will pay your fee.'

The Pied Piper started to blow a tune on his pipe. It was strange and sweet, and slowly all the rats began to appear from all the houses and sheds. He started to walk away from the town and the rats followed him. He led them to the edge of a cliff and all the rats disappeared. He returned to the Mayor and asked for his fee, but the Mayor refused to pay him and said that he should be on his way.

The Piper turned and started to play another tune, again sweet and strange, and all the children of the town rushed out to follow him along the valley. As they came near the cliff, the rock opened and all the children danced inside. All except one child who was lame and could not walk fast enough.

The Pied Piper went on his way and the people of Hamelin learned a big lesson.

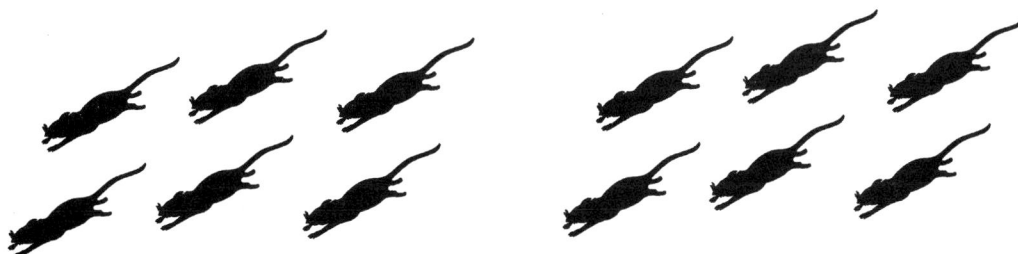

Worksheet 4.1
Spider Glove Puppets

You will need: fabric or wool gloves, white glue, sequins, buttons, pipe-cleaners, needle and thread, coloured and black wool, felt scraps.

1 Choose a knitted glove or a fabric one – make sure it fits! Choose what colour spider you want, but realistic colours are usually the most scary.

2 Put on the glove and play with it; make it 'slither and scuttle, creep and crawl, weave and writhe' before deciding how to decorate it.

3 Choose buttons (sewing), sequins (sticking), scraps (sticking) to make large round eyes, and a mouth (what shape?)

4 Put on the glove and play with it again and decide what else you need to define the character. Maybe 'hair'?

5 Small bunches of wool can create hair.

6 Spiders have 2–8 eyes. Add extra eyes.

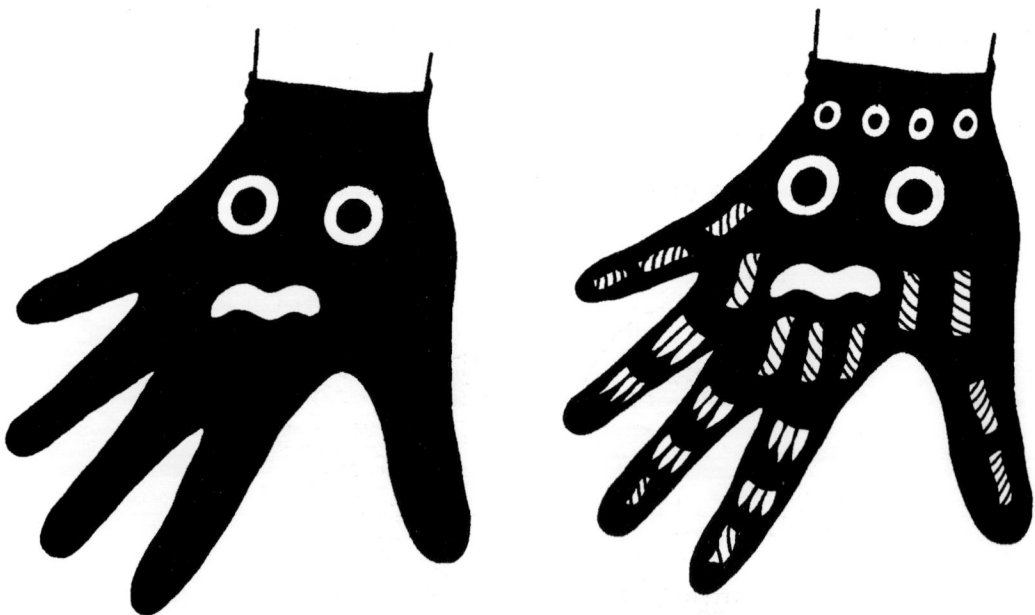

Worksheet 4.2
Rat Sock Puppet

You will need: odd socks in black or grey, scraps of felt or fur fabric, white glue, thick string or twine, round black buttons, darning needle and white wool.

1 Examine the sock and see where you can attach the various extra features. Make a decision whether you are sewing or sticking.

2 Choose round shiny buttons and sew them on for eyes, or cut out felt circles and stick them on.

3 Use the white wool to sew two teeth or cut them from white paper and stick them on.

4 Cut small triangles from fur fabric or felt and sew either side to make ears. Otherwise, stick the felt with white glue.

5 The thick string can be used for the rat's tail.

Spend some time practising the movements of the rat and, if working with a class, practise a group of rats being able to move together.

Think of different rat stories and rhymes that you can play with, for example:

• This is the house that Jack built: this is the rat that ate the malt that lay in the house that Jack built.

• There was a crooked man, who walked a crooked mile, who found a crooked sixpence, beside a crooked stile. He bought a crooked cat, that caught a crooked rat, and they all lived together, in a little crooked house.

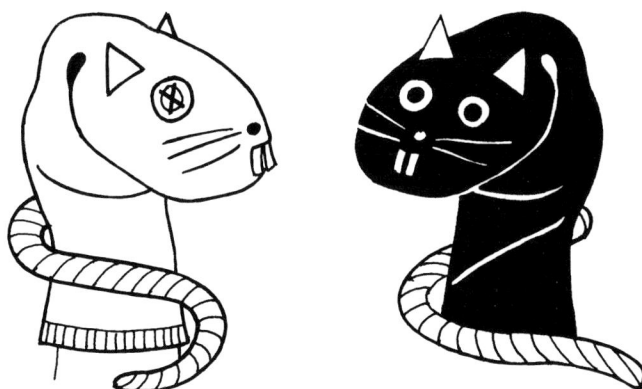

Worksheet 4.3
Moving Mouth Sock Puppets

Version 1

You will need: glue, cardboard buttons, red paper felt or fabric, wool, socks, felt pen.

1 Cut an oval of cardboard which you can paint red with a felt pen, fold in half.

2 Insert the cardboard on top of the sock between your thumb and fingers.

3 You now have a moveable mouth.

4 Complete features with buttons, wool, glue in red tongue.

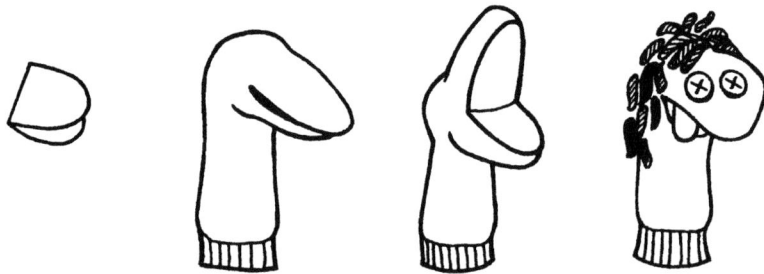

Version 2

1 Cut an oval of cardboard no wider than your sock. Fold in half.

2 Turn the sock inside out. Flatten it so that the seam runs from side to side.

3 Coat the inside fold of the cardboard with glue. Press the sock into the fold as shown. Leave the glue to dry.

4 Turn the sock right side out, and pull it back over the cardboard until the puppet has a smiling mouth.

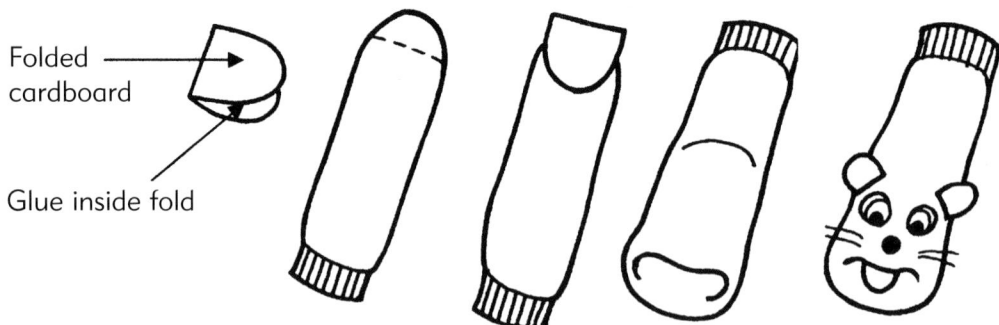

Folded cardboard

Glue inside fold

Worksheet 4.4
Creating Stories for your Puppets

Think about a story for the characters of the sock puppets.
What puppets have you made?

_____

_____

_____

_____

Where do they live?
What are their names and ages?
Do they know each other?
Who has a story to tell?

Let each puppet create their own story that involves the
other puppets.
Write your story here:

_____

_____

_____

_____

_____

_____

_____

_____

You can continue your story on the back of this sheet.

CHAPTER 5

Stick Puppets

A Stick is not just a Stick

WE HAVE TALKED IN PREVIOUS CHAPTERS about how our fingers and hands can become puppets in many different ways. If we just place a stick in our hand – perhaps a coffee stick when we have a large cappuccino – we have the beginnings of a puppet. The stick is an extension of our hand, and once we stick on a face, we have a puppet. Always save the sticks you get in cafés and most managers will give you a bundle if they know it is for 'special needs' work.

I like to use natural pieces of wood that have been stripped of bark and then smoothed: all the different trees have different textures. I have a stick-maker who uses pieces that have been blown off trees: oak, yew, beech, willow and rowan. These are the sticks I use for various exercises but I do not use these sticks for making the puppets. This is because the sticks are mini-works of art and take a long time to make – I even have to wait for the wood to be blown down in a storm!

You may have to use plastic batons (yuk!) but why not use wooden spoons? The wood is smooth and some spoons have relatively small heads. You can also use pieces of dowel rod (such as is used to make the backs of chairs or the sides of cots); they are round and smooth and can be easily held. A friendly local wood supplier may well have off-cuts. I have also obtained some from a second-hand chair store where the chairs had damaged seats and could not be repaired. The ideal length of the dowelling should be 30 cms (12 inches) or two pencil lengths.

Movement and Voice Warm Ups

Just as we have had exercises for warming up the body and especially the hands and voice for puppet work, there are exercises we can do with our sticks to anticipate stick puppet work. You will have your own rules regarding health and safety and the use of sticks.

- Have a stick in each hand and pretend to 'conduct' some lively music. This exercise develops the whole of the upper body and assists with coordination (for music suggestions see Chapter 11, p195).
- Choose more relaxed music and conduct it in a slower more soothing way.
- Allow one person to conduct and get everyone else to play imaginary musical instruments. Have music playing in the background.
- Invite people to go into pairs: one person is a musician and the other is a musical instrument.
- Repeat any of the above exercises and use your voice to make the sound of the instrument.
- Remember that for all brass and wind instruments you need plenty of breath. Practise deep breathing exercises in which the breath goes right down into your diaphragm. Practise breathing in, holding your breath and then slowly breathing out through your mouth.

Miming with Sticks to Develop the Imagination

- Sit in a circle and place one stick in the centre and invite people to use the stick as different things: for example, a boat paddle, a kitchen whisk, a violin bow, a banana.
- With a partner, use one stick (or two) to create a scene in which the stick is something other than a stick (non-verbally).
- Use a stick (or two) to beat out a rhythm (as if they are drumsticks) and move to the rhythm.
- Combine everyone's rhythms into an integrated piece: create movement or dance to go with the rhythm.

- Try to balance your stick on the end of your finger and then move round the room.
- Have an imaginary stick on the end of your finger or on your chin, and create the illusion that you are balancing it (keep your eyes fixed on the stick).
- If you do not have safe sticks, then manipulate an imaginary stick and blow up an imaginary balloon and pat the balloon to and from a partner.
- Go to a small river bridge and play 'Pooh-sticks' with any suitable sticks you can find: drop them in the water on one side of the bridge – then run over to see them appear on the other side.

Household Puppets

The most simple stick puppets can be made from household articles and elaborated with glued-on decorations. Wooden spoons, pegs, mops, pan scrubbers and brushes can take on a whole new life once you see their potential as puppet characters. They are easy and inexpensive to acquire and do not need preparation of the wood (although it is as well to check for any splinters). Wooden 'dolly' pegs are getting more difficult to find, as there is more and more availability of plastic pegs. However, I find that many small town hardware stores do still stock them.

Take a few moments to look around your own kitchen or the kitchen at work or your local hardware store and allow your imagination to run riot! The potential for puppetry within the home through a range of objects that can be found in the kitchen, the bathroom and the cleaning cupboard are endless.

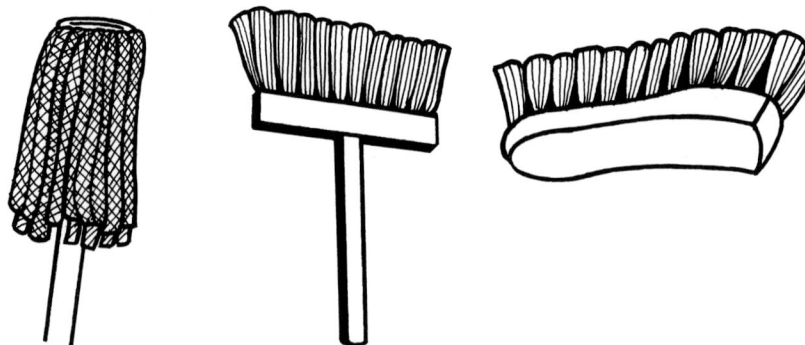

- Turn the large brushes and mops upside down and let them have a conversation with each other.
- Use hand brushes and saucepan brushes in a similar way: the bristles become very realistic hair.
- What electrical things are there in the house that might become animated (think of the Noo-Noo vacuum cleaner in Teletubbies): a kettle, a juicer, or a blender. What voices or sounds would they make?
- Create the movement, sound and then a character for a pop-up toaster: there are double toasters and there are multiple toasters.
- Remember 'The Toothbrush Song' by Max Bygraves? Probably only if you are over forty! Many of the adults you work with will recall this silly song about a pink and a blue toothbrush that want to get married and share the same toothpaste. Use it as a stimulus to develop toothbrush ideas. Toothbrushes can make very good puppets, and they are cheap to purchase or given away free in hotels and on aeroplanes.
- I would probably hesitate to use everything in the bathroom for animation as I think loo conversation would lend itself to crudity but maybe I am being old-fashioned. However a conversation through showerheads could be great fun!

Once you bring inanimate objects to life you have a whole puppet theatre. You can encourage members of your group to do the same and see what ideas they have for making puppets. When you first make suggestions, try asking the group what objects in their kitchen could become a character in a story; let the idea for puppets come afterwards. They are likely to think this is very silly, but I feel you can all join in the fun.

Some adults may need reminding that many cartoons are based on objects acquiring a life; think of films such as *The Sorcerer's Apprentice, The Mask, Toy Story, Harry Potter, Fantasia, Lord of the Rings* or *High Society* where objects and plants become animated. Remember the trees in *Lord of the Rings*? Or the broomsticks in *The Sorcerer's Apprentice*?

Sounds and Dialogue

You can use the above examples to 'get people going' but try to encourage them to think of their own ideas, and you can make suggestions without imposing them. For example:

- Think of all the 'rings and pings' in the house and make up a group tune: for example there are kitchen ringers, the microwave, door bells, mobile phones, alarm clocks.
- Create a conversation between different messages that we hear on answer machines.
- Have a discussion about the types of music we have to listen to when we are waiting for someone to answer us.
- Create a scene where people can answer back to all the messages they hear when trying to call their bank or electricity and gas company.

There is a good example of this in the radio play 'If you're Glad, I'll be Frank' by Tom Stoppard (1976). In the play, a bus driver is desperate to talk to his estranged wife and is convinced that it is her voice on the speaking clock when he dials up to find out the time. You could use scenes from the play to encourage your group to think of other ideas.

Making Scripts from Newspapers and Catalogues

What might the puppets say?

There are many lines and phrases in advertisements in magazines and catalogues that suggest the product can speak! Germs, teabags and yoghurt all express themselves through words and sounds. Once people are aware of this they will make a connection with the idea of a puppet.

- Use old newspapers, catalogues and magazines and encourage people to cut out 'selling lines' from advertisements. Use these lines to create a scene.

- You can also use lines and phrases to make a story or a poem. For many people it is easier and less daunting to use other people's words.
- Headlines from newspapers can also be used to make a poem or a story or a scene.

Out and About: Further Inspiration for Puppets

The popular revival of *Thomas the Tank Engine* stories, now being developed by the Reverend Awdry's family, is another example of an object becoming 'live'. A clergyman who was trying to entertain his son while he was ill with scarlet fever first wrote these children's stories in 1945. His son insisted on the stories being repeated accurately so his father wrote them down. The rest, as they say, is history and Thomas is now a very big business. You only have to look at the faces on the front of the engines and imagine them as puppet faces on a stick.

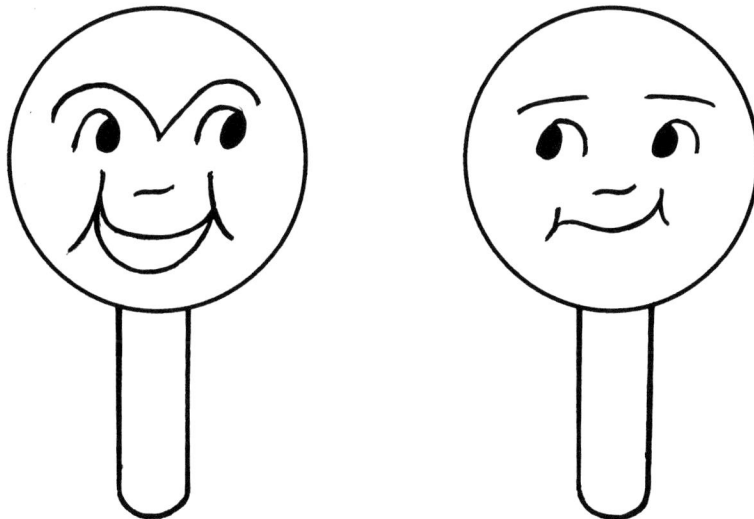

Recently I saw a local bus with a destination board that read, 'I'm sorry, I am not in service'. Since when did a bus express regret? What is wrong with the old sign, 'Not in Service'? However for our purposes it is ideal because it gives an example of an inanimate object expressing something! The bus has almost become a puppet!

- Encourage people to look at the front of cars, lorries, buses, and see if they have 'expressions': look at these in reality or in advertisements. Create a conversation between two contrasting vehicles: a Mini and a lorry; a bus and a limousine, for example.
- Follow through similar ideas with different types of boats or trains, aeroplanes or space rockets.
- Cut out a picture of a vehicle, stick it on card, glue a stick on the back and you have a simple puppet.

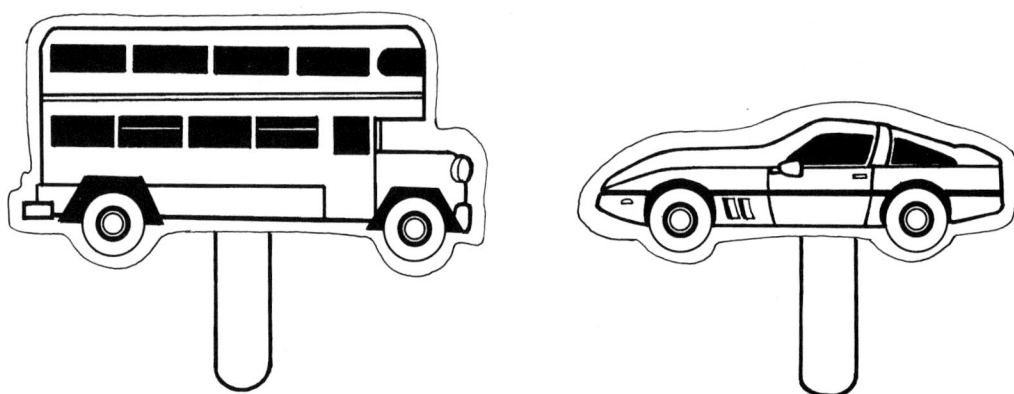

Fun at the Garden and Discount Shop

We seem to be buying more and more decorations to place in the garden or to stick in our plant pots. Many of them will only last for a few weeks after extreme weather – both sun and storms. However, these decorations are ideal for stick puppet work. Most of them are made on wooden sticks, so check for splinters; others have a stick made of metal. These are less easy to hold as the metal is very narrow, but they can be tied to a (wooden) stick.

Naturally, it is important to be careful when using bare metal with a group who may be volatile or aggressive.

- Take time to explore your garden shop and see just how many things can be used as puppets.
- You will also want to purchase bundles of garden stakes (the ones to which we tie pot plants or garden plants) for use with various stick puppets.
- Choose a selection of butterflies and birds, they are usually attached by a small spring and therefore 'wobble'. Use them as stick puppets and create conversations and scenes.
- Create scenery or additional characters through the various flowers on sticks, such as sunflowers.
- You can also make simple sunflowers and stick them onto coffee or garden sticks.

How to Make the Puppets

Let's get on to the puppets. There are a variety of stock puppets that can be made quite easily. My suggestions here include: Paper Plate Puppet, Newspaper Heads, and Wooden Spoon Puppets. The basic stick puppet is a stick with a face. The following are ideas for the simplest ones you can make, and they only involve one stick and are easy to hold. However, do remember that people's arms can tire, especially people with disabilities, so puppets can 'talk' with the arm resting on a table or chair back. For some people sitting around a table gives security, and if possible make it a round table for greater communication.

Materials needed

A selection of sticks that include: garden sticks (take care of splinters), coffee and lolly sticks; large and small paper plates; newspapers; an assortment of wooden spoons; wood glue and white glue; long pins; masking tape; balls of wool, string, raffia; strips of paper; pipe cleaners; scraps of material including pieces that are 30 cms (12 inches) square; coloured pens; sequins, buttons and feathers.

Paper Plates

- Create a face on a paper plate and glue or tape a stick to the back; you can suggest random faces, or the face can be for a specific story, such as 'The Birth of Athena' (see Worksheet 5.2).
- Some people cannot grasp the idea of drawing just the head and will draw a head and body: that is fine and should not be challenged.
- Let the puppets talk to each other in pairs and then in small groups.
- In a small group create a puppet play that can tell a story, and perhaps perform it to the other groups.
- The paper plates can also become masks (see Chapter 7).

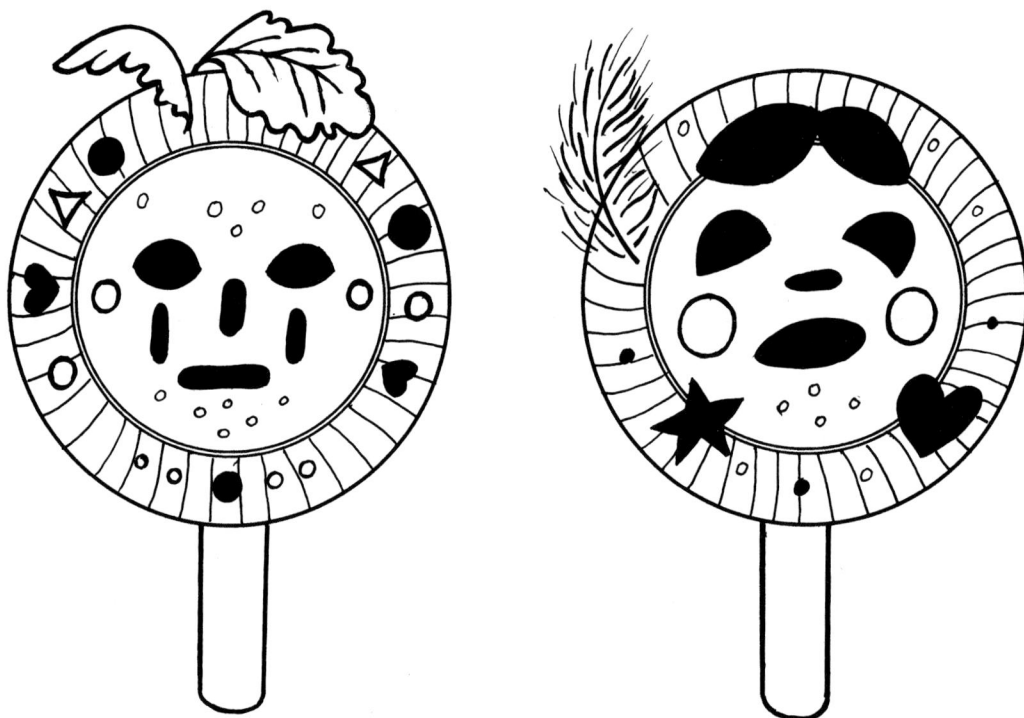

Newspaper Heads

- Scrunch up a ball of newspaper somewhere between the size of a ping-pong ball and a tennis ball.
- Shape it by using strips of masking tape to hold the newspaper and to mould the features.

- Decide on the character and create the features, either by sticking on scraps of material or by drawing with the coloured pens.
- Make hair from wool, or string, or strips of paper or draw the hair with coloured pens.
- Use wood glue to attach the newspaper head to the stick.
- You now have a stick puppet that is quite unique.
- Explore the possibilities of your puppet as a character, experiment with different voices.
- Work with a partner to dramatise a scene or to tell a story.
- Resist the temptation to make puppets and then put them on the walls as decorations: puppets are meant to be brought to life with movement, voice and stories.

Wooden Spoons

Spoons give us a puppet shape with an oval head and a stick handle. They are smooth and easy to grasp (and should satisfy health and safety requirements). Some spoons are coated and do not take paint easily so check before you buy. Car boot sales and jumble sales sometimes have a box of kitchen items that include spoons and other wooden items.

Each person should be given a wooden spoon. Remember that once they are painted the features cannot be rubbed out, so encourage people to develop their ideas first – perhaps making sketches of the type of face they would like to create. People need to decide if they want a fuller face on the back of the spoon or a slightly convex face by using the front. However, it is possible to change the shape of the head with newspaper and masking tape. You can 'fill in' one side to make the whole head symmetric.

- Think of a fairy-tale character and the expression they might have on their face.
- Draw it on the spoon with coloured pens.
- Make hair and stick it on.
- Create the idea of a costume: maybe a collar or a bow-tie.
- Dramatise the story with all the puppets.

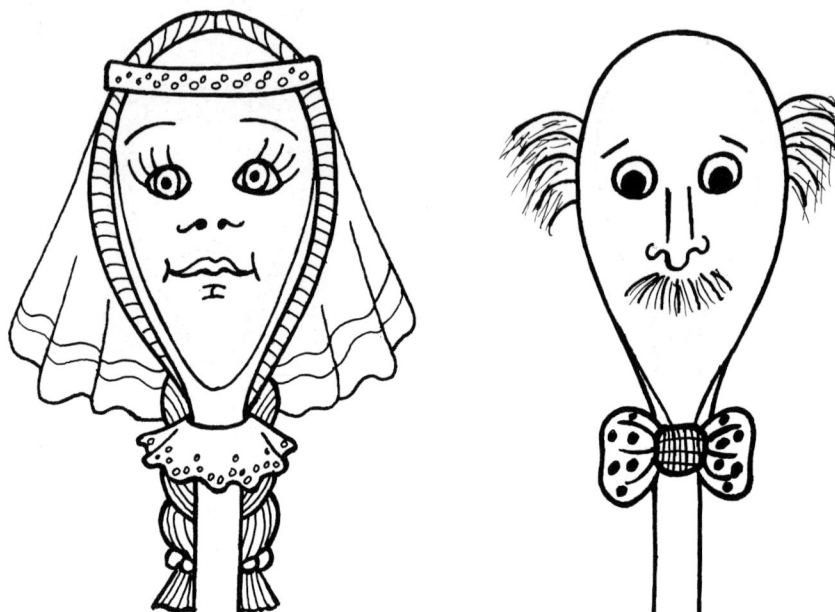

More complex spoons
- A spoon puppet can also be dressed in costumes, but it needs the addition of shoulders in order for the material to 'hang' correctly.
- Make a small ball of newspaper that you can wrap around the spoon handle roughly a finger length below the face (finger = 2 finger joints down on first finger). Secure it with masking tape, or better still, with wood glue.
- Once you have shoulders, you can hang a simple costume: a cape or a shawl, a dress or a shirt. Finish the costume by sticking or sewing on sequins, buttons, feathers.
- Create a head-covering: a shawl, a bonnet, a hat, a cap, a witches' hat, a crown. Secure it firmly with glue or a long pin.
- Place your puppet and head on a piece of material and make sure that the shoulders and the costume are in proportion to the puppet as a whole.
- Material can be sewn or stuck with glue. Secure it well on the shoulders, otherwise you will find that the head can move in one direction and the body in another!
- You could also cover pipe cleaners and twist them round to make arms
- If you have arms, then your puppet can have something to carry: an umbrella, a bag, a stick.

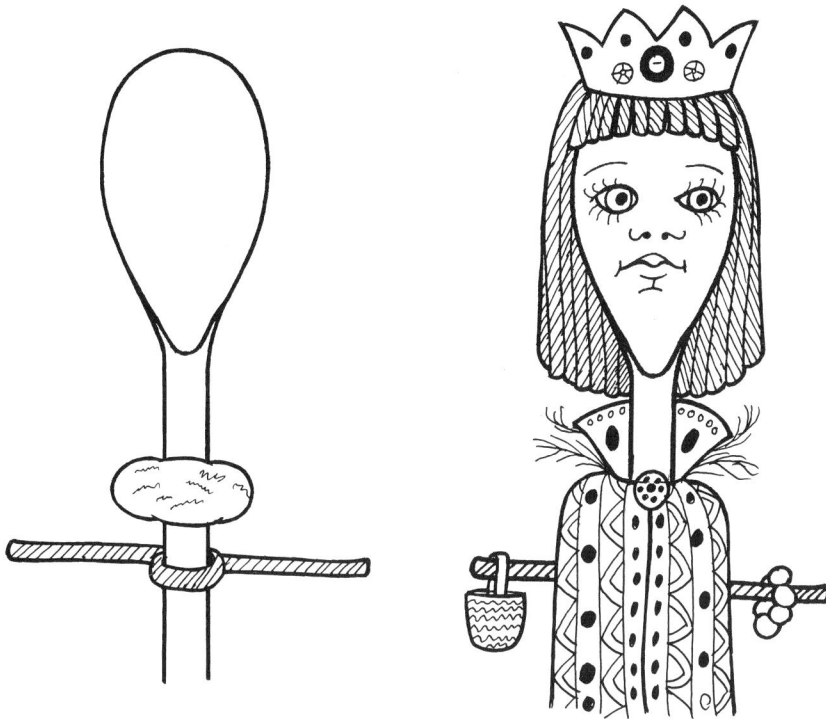

- Try making up your own story with all the characters
- If you are working with adults, maybe they could create a puppet show for a group of children.

Enacting Stories with Simple Stick Puppets

The following stories can be enacted with any of the basic stick puppets in this chapter. They can all be adapted to different characters and scenery can be stuck onto a stick as well. The instructions are on Worksheets 5.1 and 5.2.

The Story of the Thunder Bird

To enact this story you will need to make the following puppets:

- Snails: draw on card, cut them out and secure to small sticks.
- Poor man with raggedy clothes: follow instruction for the one-stick puppet.
- Thunder bird: follow the instructions on Worksheet 5.1.
- Elementals: water, fire, thunder, lightning, rain. Follow instructions from shadow theatre puppets in Chapter 6.

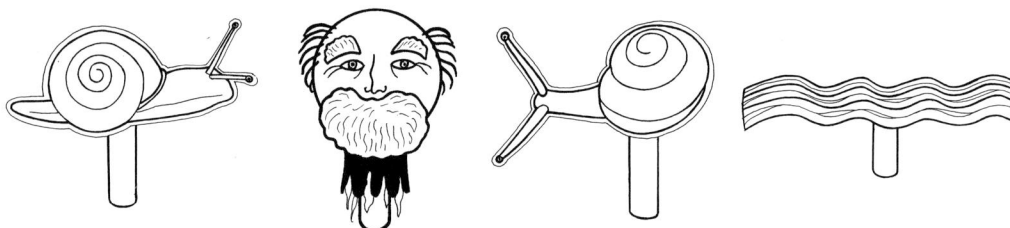

The Story

In a land far away, a poor man was fishing for snails.

Every time he put a snail on the bank, the thunder bird took it away into the forest and put it on the fire at the edge of the forest. The poor man could see smoke rising from the thunder bird's fire and thought that if he could have fire, he could cook his snails instead of eating them raw.

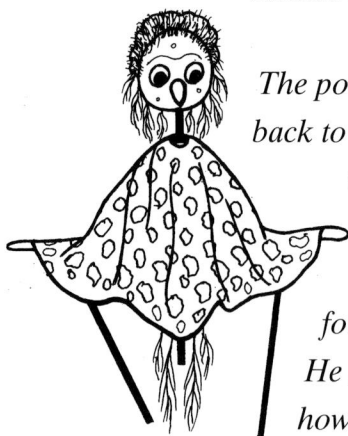

The poor man decided to follow the thunder bird back to the forest, and watched while he was cooking the snails and eating them. The smell was delicious. The bird flew away looking for more food to cook and the poor man crept forward and took the fire sticks away with him. He returned to his village and showed everyone how they could cook their food on the fire.

The thunder bird was angry and beat his wings, and a great storm blew up. There was great thunder and lightning and the rains came and put out the fire. The poor man had kept some fire inside an earthenware pot that did not get put out by the rains.

The villagers were able to cook their food, but every time they heard thunder, they knew that the thunder bird was still angry because the poor man had taken the fire to cook his snails.

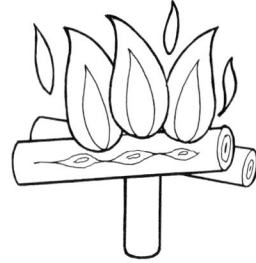

The Birth of Athena – A Stick Puppet Play

You will need to make the following puppets for this story:

- Athena
- Zeus
- Hephaestus
- Metis
- Zeus' parents

In ancient Greece, Zeus had several relationships with many of the great goddesses. But of course he was king of the gods and could do whatever he wanted – well, almost.

For some time Zeus was a consort of Metis who was considered wise, and able to foretell the future.

The parents of Zeus were most concerned. They predicted that Metis would have twins; the daughter would give him no cause for concern but the boy twin would be a danger to Zeus. He would become more powerful and stronger than the king of the gods himself.

Zeus copied what his father had done and swallowed his children. Zeus swallowed Metis who was already pregnant and rested more easily now that he had control of any future children.

Zeus was out walking and developed as big a headache as he had ever experienced in his life. He was in terrible pain.

Hephaestus, his adult child who was lame, took a huge and sharp axe and split his father's forehead open. Athena was born out of her father's forehead, fully grown and fully armed. She arrived with a battle cry!

Athena the warrior goddess had arrived, and would later found the city of Athens.

Worksheet 5.1
The Story of the Thunder Bird

To make three stick puppets you will need: three garden sticks, newspapers, masking tape, wood and white glue, feathers, scraps of materials, black pen.

1 Create an oval-shaped body from newspaper and wood, then glue it to one stick, a third of the way down.

2 Take a piece of material in the colour you would like for your bird, 30 cms (12 inches) square. Fold it in four and cut a small circle at the point and then place it on the 'body'. One point will hang down in front, one behind, and one on each side.

3 The other two sticks need to be tied to each of the material side points. Place the stick under the material and wind it round and round with wool.

4 Create the head and the beak from another ball of newspaper and use masking tape to sculpt the bird's head with a beak. You may want to stick on an extra piece of paper for the beak. Draw or stick on the eyes. Use feathers to stick on the back of the head. Glue the head onto the stick and stick more feathers on the body. Your bird is now complete.

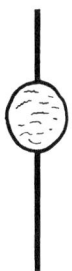
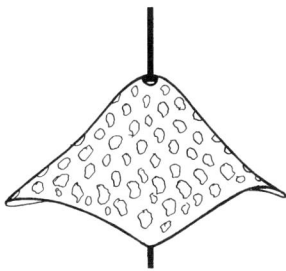
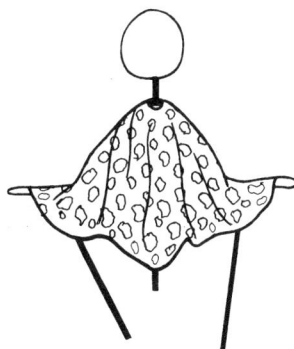
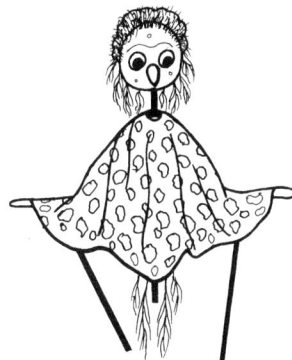

1   2   3   4

Speechmark P This page may be photocopied for instructional use only. *Creative Puppetry with Children & Adults* © Sue Jennings 2008

Worksheet S.2
The Birth of Athena –
A Stick Puppet Play

Members of the group can each make a puppet for the story. They can either create simple stick puppets, or be really daring and create the three stick puppets for the main characters.

Photocopy the pictures below, enlarge them on to card, cut them out and stick them to small coffee sticks. You can create different additional characters for your play if you wish.

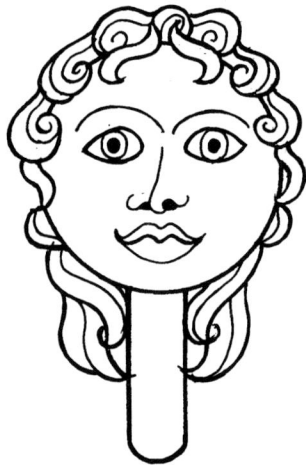
Athena

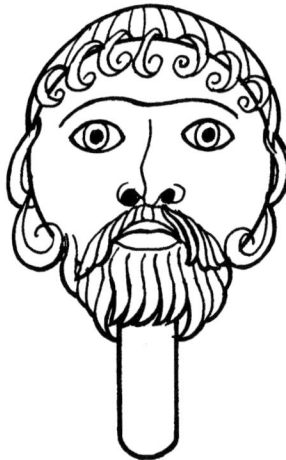
Zeus

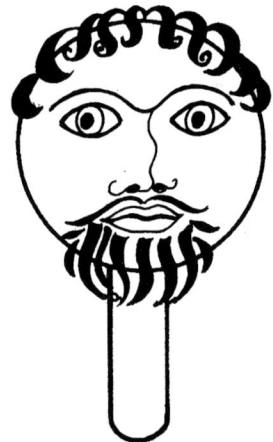
Hephaestus

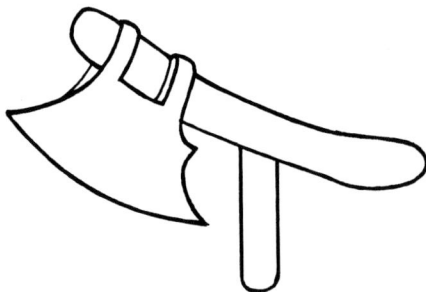

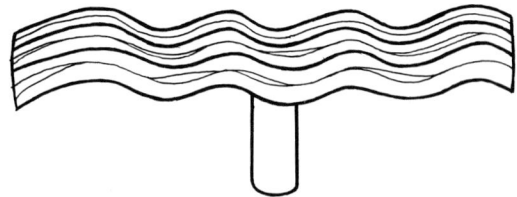

In groups of five find different ways to tell or enact the story.

CHAPTER 6

Shadow Puppets

S HADOW PUPPETS HAVE A VERY ANCIENT HISTORY that we touched on earlier and it seems that of all the puppet traditions, it is the shadow puppet that has proved most flexible and adaptable. In this chapter we shall consider both ancient stories using puppets and more contemporary tales than can become puppet plays.

Shadow Hands

The simplest of shadow puppets can be made with our own hands as they throw a shadow on the wall. Hand warm-ups from Chapters 2 and 3 are very useful before we begin our shadow work.

Have a light source that will throw shadows onto a light wall and encourage people to experiment. The simplest shadow puppet is probably a duck created by all the fingers being very flat, the knuckles being the dome of the head and the thumb forming the beak.

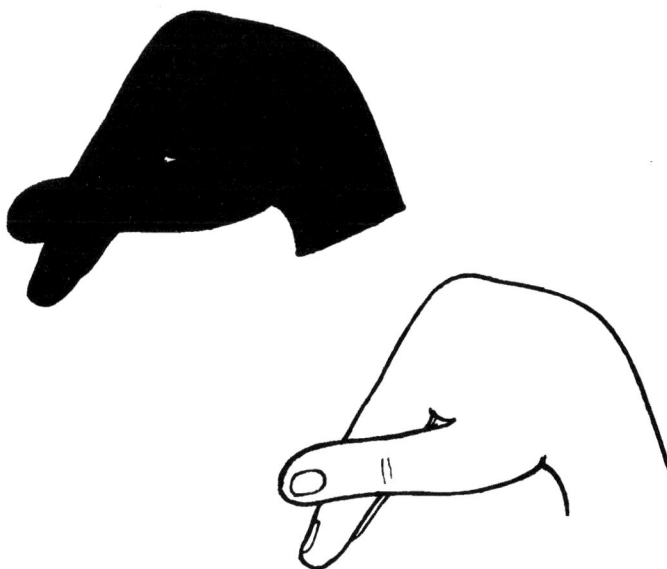

Duck shapes

You can also make a wolf by again making the fingers flat and this time using the thumb to create the ear:

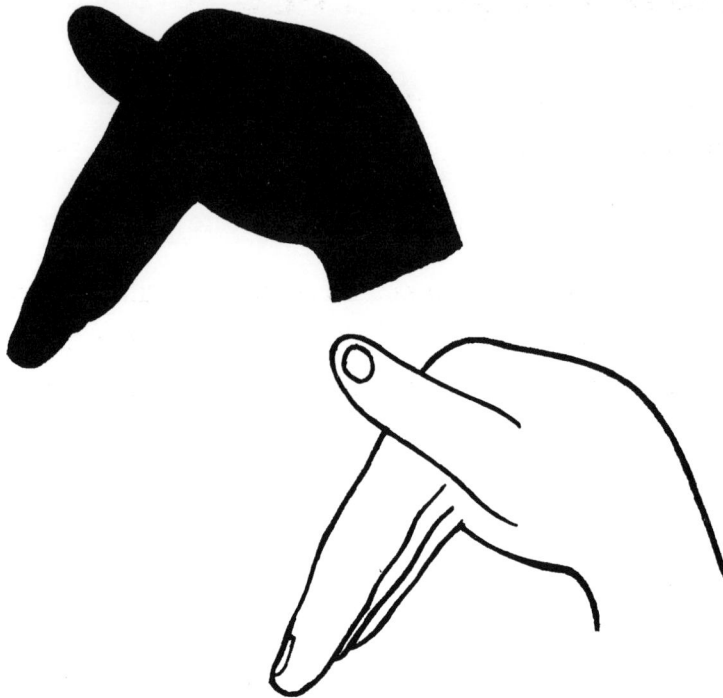

A wolf

You can then make a simple story about the duck and the wolf, in pairs, with each person making one shadow hand puppet.

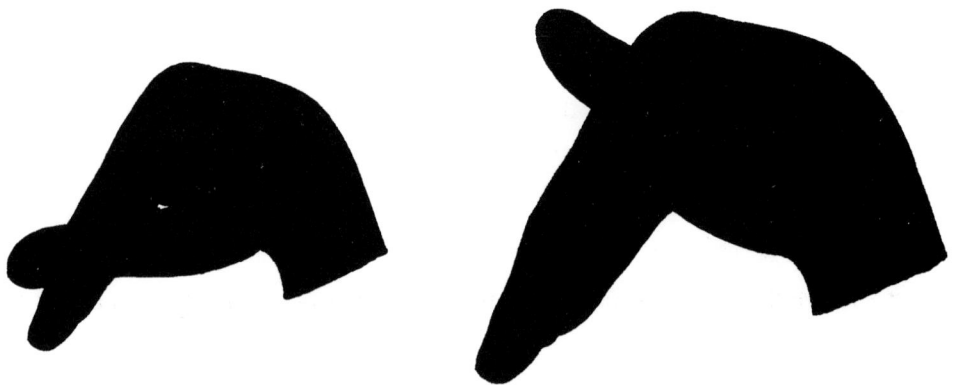

Creating a Shadow Puppet Theatre

You will need: thick card or cardboard, pencils, strong tape, small sticks, a white sheet, a light source (bulb or torch), two upright supports such as lamp stands.

Encourage people to draw an outline of a person onto thick card. You can use old boxes, as long as they are not plastic coated. The person can be anyone, but make it at least 20 cms (8 inches) tall. Cut it out and use strong tape to attach a small stick on the back – at right angles.

You may want to experiment yourself with the shadow puppet before trying it with your group or class.

Tie a white sheet across two light stands (or suitable supports) to make a screen. Have a single light behind the screen. Although traditionally candles would have been used as the light source, make sure the light bulb is safe. For example you can use a small strip light or one of the low wattage safety bulbs. A very powerful torch would do but then batteries will be an expense!

When you have tested the screen, let some of the group be audience and some manipulate their puppets across the screen. They can move across the screen or move into the background to suggest leaving the scene. Remember that features are not seen, only outlines, so a clear silhouette is essential.

With a group of children you may want to try animal silhouettes that they free draw. Encourage free drawing in the early stages; tracing can come later.

When you have practised with these simple puppets and maybe improvised short stories and plays, you can move onto a story and design the puppets especially for enacting it in a shadow theatre.

The Story of the Poisoned Apple

The following story is ideal for telling through shadow puppets because it has straightforward characters and simple staging. Let's tell the story first:

In the days of King Arthur, Morgana le Fay wanted to discredit Arthur as she was very jealous of his queen, Guinevere. She put poison into an apple and placed it into a fruit bowl on the Round Table. The knights were sitting round the table having their lunch and chatting about their latest adventures.

Queen Guinevere saw the beautiful apple and was about to eat it when she noticed a handsome young knight sitting near her. She rubbed the apple till it shone and then leaned over and said to Sir Gaheris, the young knight, 'Please accept this apple as a sign of friendship,' and the knight replied, 'Indeed I will eat it as a sign of friendship.' The knight took only one bite and he collapsed onto the floor.

Everyone was stunned and then looked at the Queen. Another Knight, Sir Mordred, accused the Queen of poisoning Sir Gaheris. 'Don't look so innocent madam; we have all seen that you gave the apple to the knight. You have killed him and the punishment will be death.'

He went to tell King Arthur the news and then went to find the brother of Gaheris, Sir Mador.

Sir Mador shouted, 'The Queen must die for committing this murder, unless someone will defend her.' None of the knights stepped forward to defend the Queen's honour, and King Arthur looked around the assembled company with sadness. But he knew he had to obey the law.

King Arthur said, 'Is there no knight who will come forward and defend the Queen?' Nobody moved and Sir Mador issued his challenge.

*'I will wait for the challenge of a knight who is willing to defend
you, otherwise, as is stated in the law of the land, you must die.'
And he rode away to await the dual.*

*There were other knights who were as corrupt as Sir Mordred and
only wanted to bring down the Queen, inspired, of course, by
hatred of Morgana. But there were many who were very puzzled at
this conflict between the knights of the Round Table.*

*The Queen waited and waited for a knight to come forward to help
her. Her special friend Sir Gawain was a relative of the dead knight
so she could not expect his help. And her other friend, Sir Lancelot
was away fighting the wars. Nobody was willing to help her.*

*The day of the contest arrived and the crowds assembled. Sir Mador
waited and Queen Guinevere looked anxiously up and down the
crowds to see if anyone would come forward to help her. King Arthur
feared the worse. Mordred and Morgana were convinced they had
won the conflict and caused enough strife to have Guinevere killed.*

*Just then a trumpet sounded and a knight appeared to challenge
Mador. No one could see who he was. The two knights charged at
each other and Mador was felled to the ground, and the strange
knight held his sword to his throat.*

*'Proclaim the innocence of the Queen or you shall die,' he called
out. 'The Queen is innocent,' cried Sir Mador, and the strange
knight allowed him to live.*

*The stranger removed his visor and everyone stood stunned for a
moment. It was Sir Lancelot, who had returned to save the honour
of his Queen.*

*Everyone cheered, and King Arthur and Queen Guinevere were
together again'.*

This story can be performed as a play with adults or with children. It can be done in small or large groups. It is a good idea to start with simple shadow puppets and then a simple play while people get used to the differences of shadow puppets. They need a screen and a light – and a viewing audience on the other side. However I have found some remarkable 'break through' working with shadow puppets.

Preparation for the Play

To perform the play you will need someone to manipulate each puppet character and a narrator to tell the story as it goes along, with pauses for the characters to say their lines. The size of the puppet will depend on who is holding it; so it is a good idea to have a trial run with a single puppet.

The simple version

To create a shadow play of this story you will need the following puppets: King Arthur, Queen Guinevere, two knights standing (Mordred and Mador), two knights on horseback (Mador and Lancelot).

Use the illustrations on Worksheet 6.1 to trace, enlarge or copy onto thick card. The figures can be coloured in any way you wish, but remember that only the outline will show on the shadow screen. Depending on the size of the puppets, either use coffee sticks or garden sticks to manipulate them. Remember the sticks need to be attached at right angles to the puppet with either duct or parcel tape (masking tape is not strong enough).

A more complex version

As your group becomes more skilled at managing the shadow puppets you can begin to add more detail. For example, for this story you can use the outline of a castle and maybe more characters such as Morgana who places the poisoned apple, the herald with a trumpet who announces the start of the joust.

You can have a Round Table where the knights of King Arthur sit and the outline of a crowd who are watching the jousting of the two knights. You may

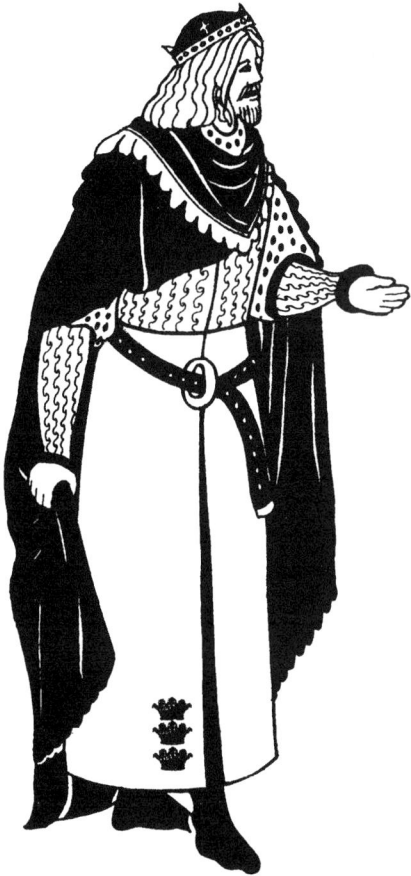

King Arthur

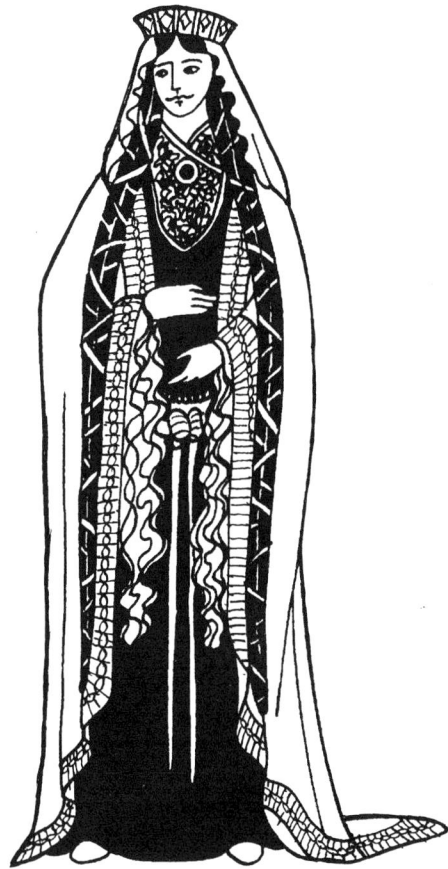

Queen Guinevere

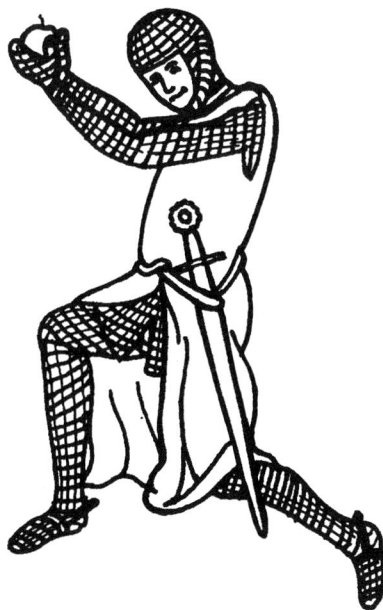

Sir Gaheris

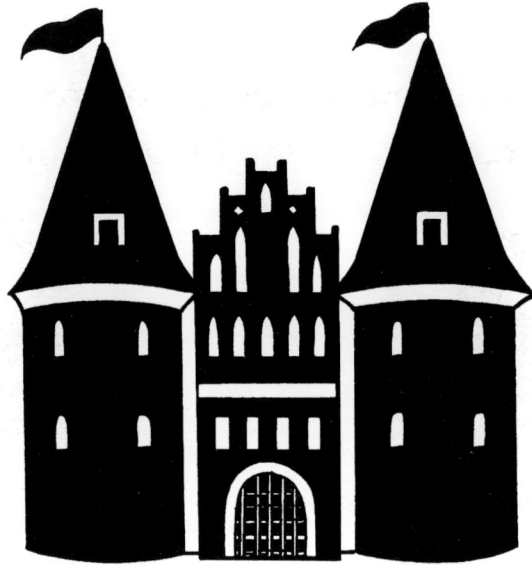

want to add puppets that represent the weather: the sun or some clouds for example.

Moving Limbs

Many traditional shadow puppets had one limb that moved and had a separate rod attached to it. Usually it was an arm that could carry something or be raised in greeting or in battle.

Putting on a Show

In this story the two knights could each carry a lance or sword in their hand, Queen Guinevere could have a handkerchief. King Arthur can also have a sword to signal the start of the combat, and the herald can have a trumpet that is lifted when he blows.

The moving arm is hinged with a brass paper clip (butterfly clip). You can set a task for people to find the best way of having a moving limb on their puppet. They can also try having a prop such as a sword or trumpet as a separate puppet so that the person has to coordinate two puppets themselves or with a partner.

Worksheet 6.1
The Story of the Poisoned Apple

Side 1

The characters below can be cut out for shadow puppets in order to tell the King Arthur story.

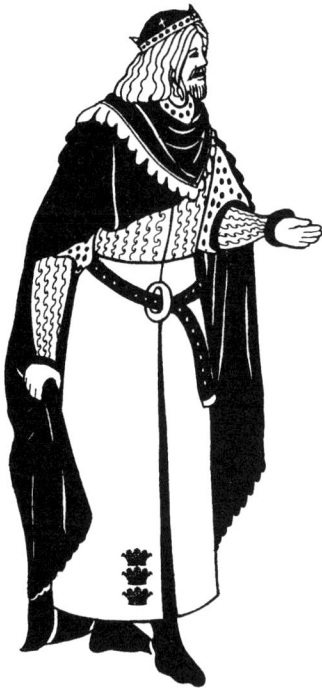

King Arthur

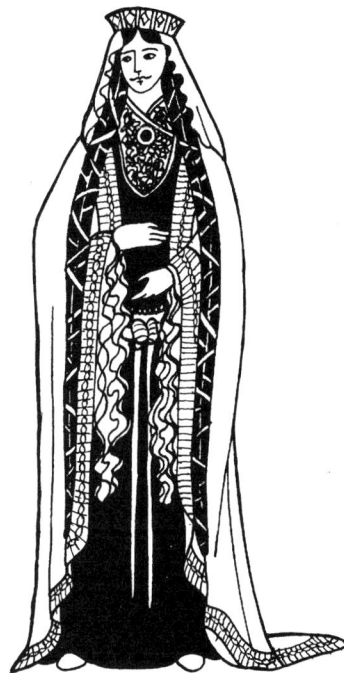

Queen Guinevere

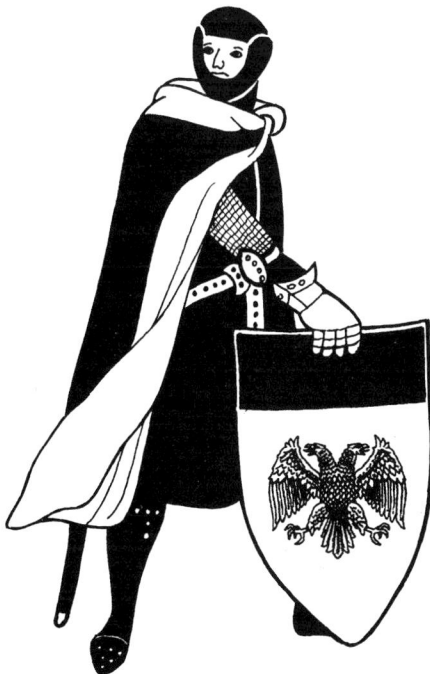

Mordred

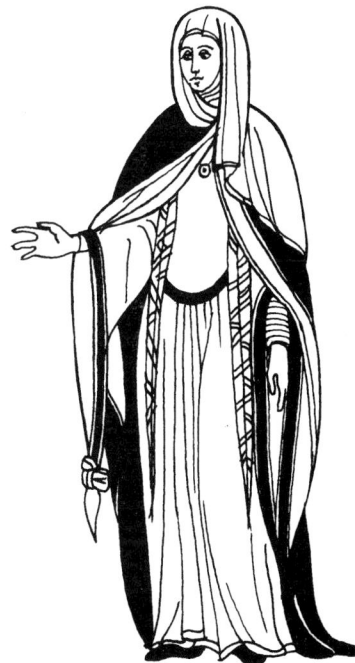

Morgana

Worksheet 6.1
The Story of the Poisoned Apple

Side 2

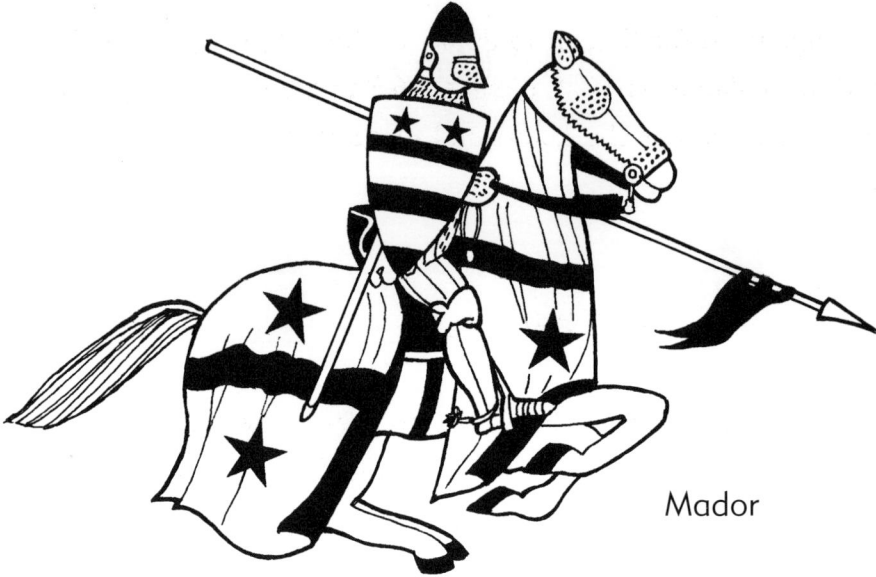

Mador

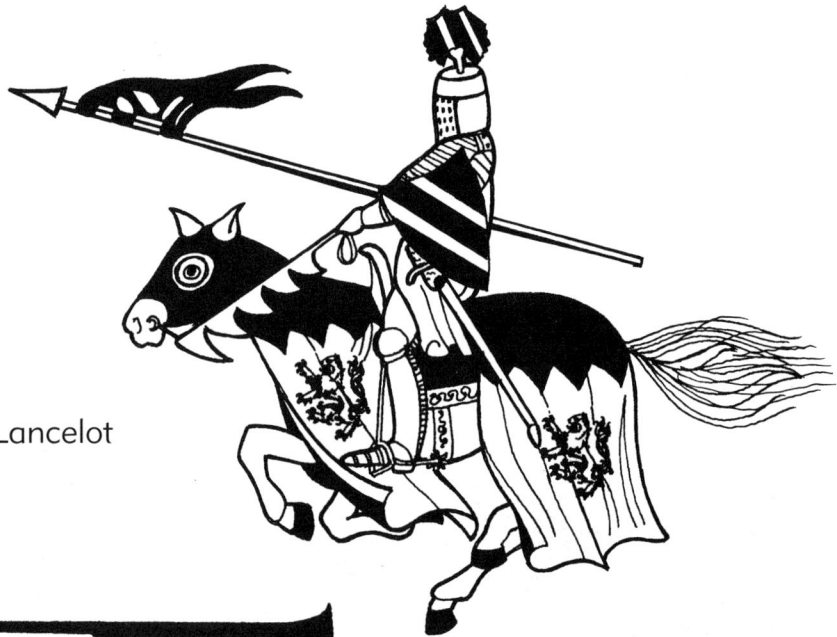

Lancelot

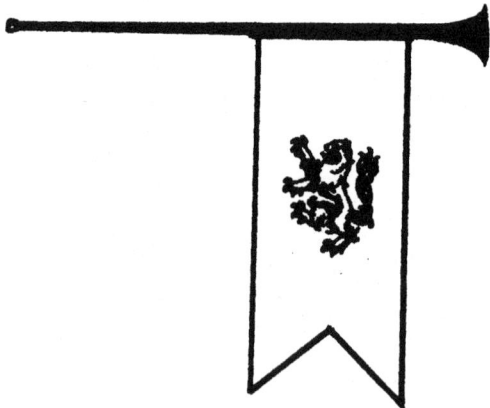

Greek Shadow Puppets

The Greeks are renowned for their traditional shadow puppet plays which use puppets with articulated parts. Worksheets 6.2 to 6.6 give examples of how to make the most popular characters and suggestions on creating your own plays.

The Characters

Karaghiozis (see Worksheet 6.2) is always the main character in the Greek shadow theatre tradition. He is a poor man who lives in a tumbledown house in the shadow of the Ottoman's wonderful palace.

He is always getting into scrapes and ends up being beaten, usually for stealing. He believes that he can steal for food as his family is so hungry and his long arm indicates that he is not averse to helping himself to things.

He is also quite a political character and for the Greeks represented the down-trodden poor man who had to outwit authority.

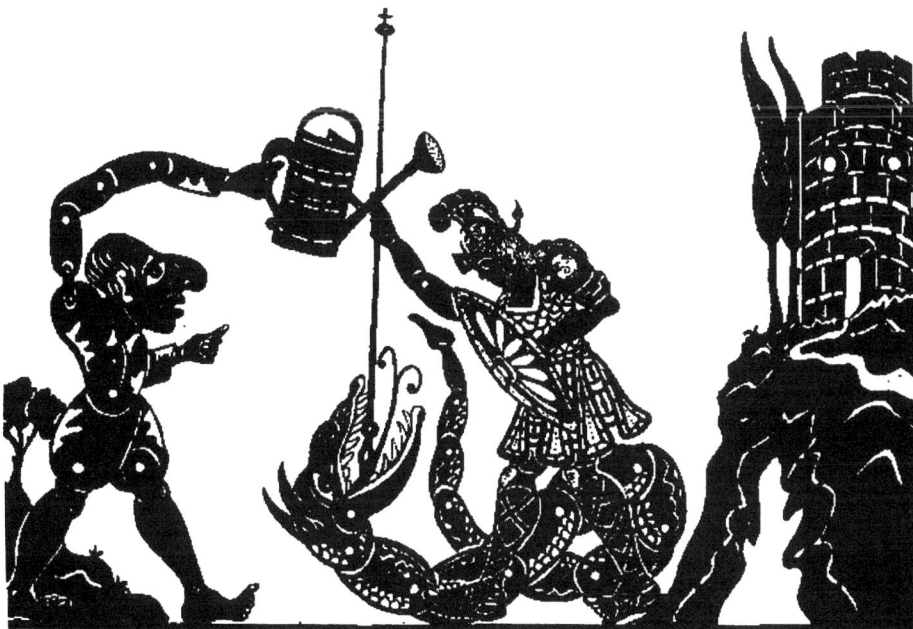

Essentially he is a trickster character who in the end gets himself out of scrapes. He is funny and wily. Do you know anyone who is like this person?

You can create stories just about him and his adventures. You can write narratives for him that someone else can read while you move the puppet. Of all the Greek shadow puppets he has the most joints and therefore is most flexible.

Baba (or Papa) Yiorgos (George) (see Worksheet 6.3) is the uncle of Karaghiozis. He is very genuine and has 'a good soul'. He lives in the village a long way from the town and is sometimes known as 'The Mountain Man' because of his simple ways.

He usually comes to town to help his nephew get out of a scrape! He also has business to conduct.

Morfonios (see Worksheet 6.5) is a very silly character, and causes the audience to laugh a lot. He has a very big head and nose.

He thinks he is handsome and boasts about his good looks. He genuinely believes he is smart, and constantly causes confusion because he lives in a fantasy world a lot of the time. He is also very greedy and tries to get things for himself. He thinks he is better than he is!

Sir Dionysios (see Worksheet 6.6) always wears a top hat. He acts as if he is from the nobility with genteel manners. He was once a prosperous aristocrat but now he has fallen on hard times. However, he still tries to keep up appearances.

All these four characters know each other and interact. They are quite distinct individuals in their own right and have well developed personalities.

Putting on a Show

Create a play as a group after discussing all the characters and decide whether it is a fairy story or some other genre; might these puppets be politicians? Or are they telling a local story from your community? All these different story styles were played out in the Greek Shadow Theatre.

Get together with all the characters and think of a scene where they can meet and interact. Who would be close to whom? Who would be helpful? Who would have the ideas?

Discuss your ideas, write your play and then rehearse it and perform it to others.

You could design a programme for the play, with coloured in pictures of the characters.

Use Worksheets 6.2 – 6.5 to create these characters. *You will need:* a rod for each character, strong tape to attach to the rod, split brass paper fasteners to create body articulations, a hole puncher.

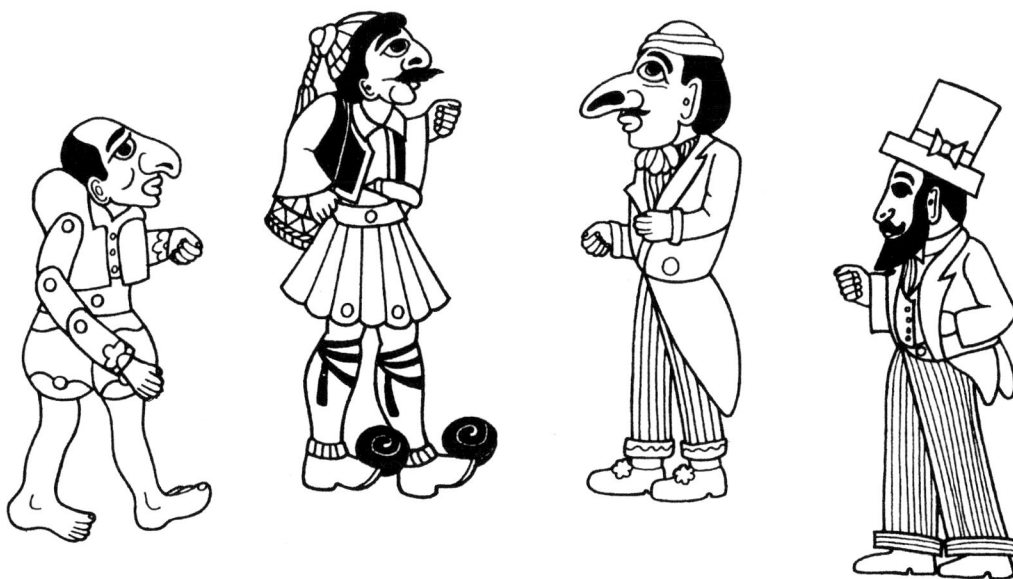

Worksheet 6.2
Greek Shadow Puppets – Karaghiozis

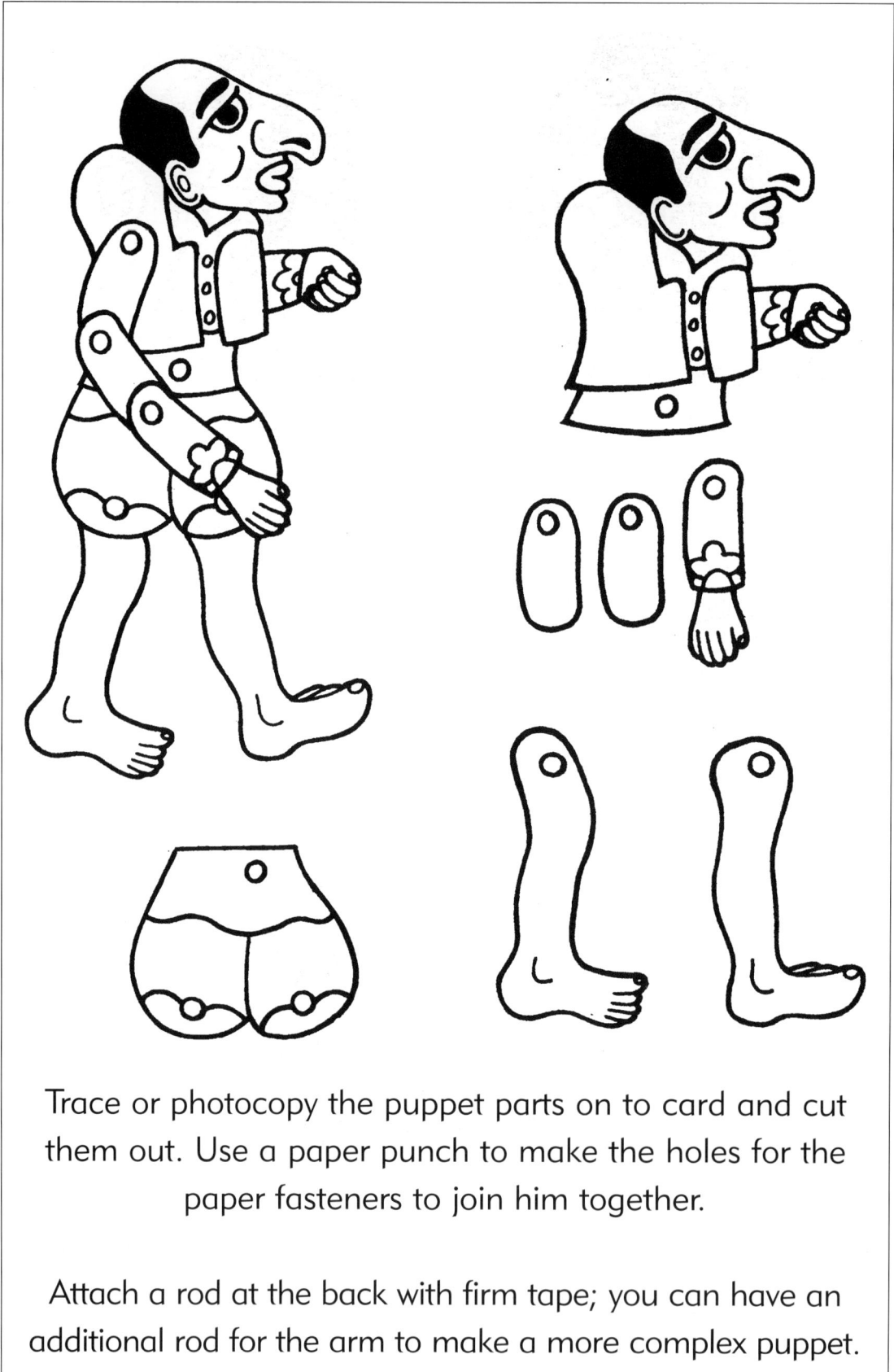

Trace or photocopy the puppet parts on to card and cut them out. Use a paper punch to make the holes for the paper fasteners to join him together.

Attach a rod at the back with firm tape; you can have an additional rod for the arm to make a more complex puppet.

Worksheet 6.3
Greek Shadow Puppets –
Baba Yiorgos

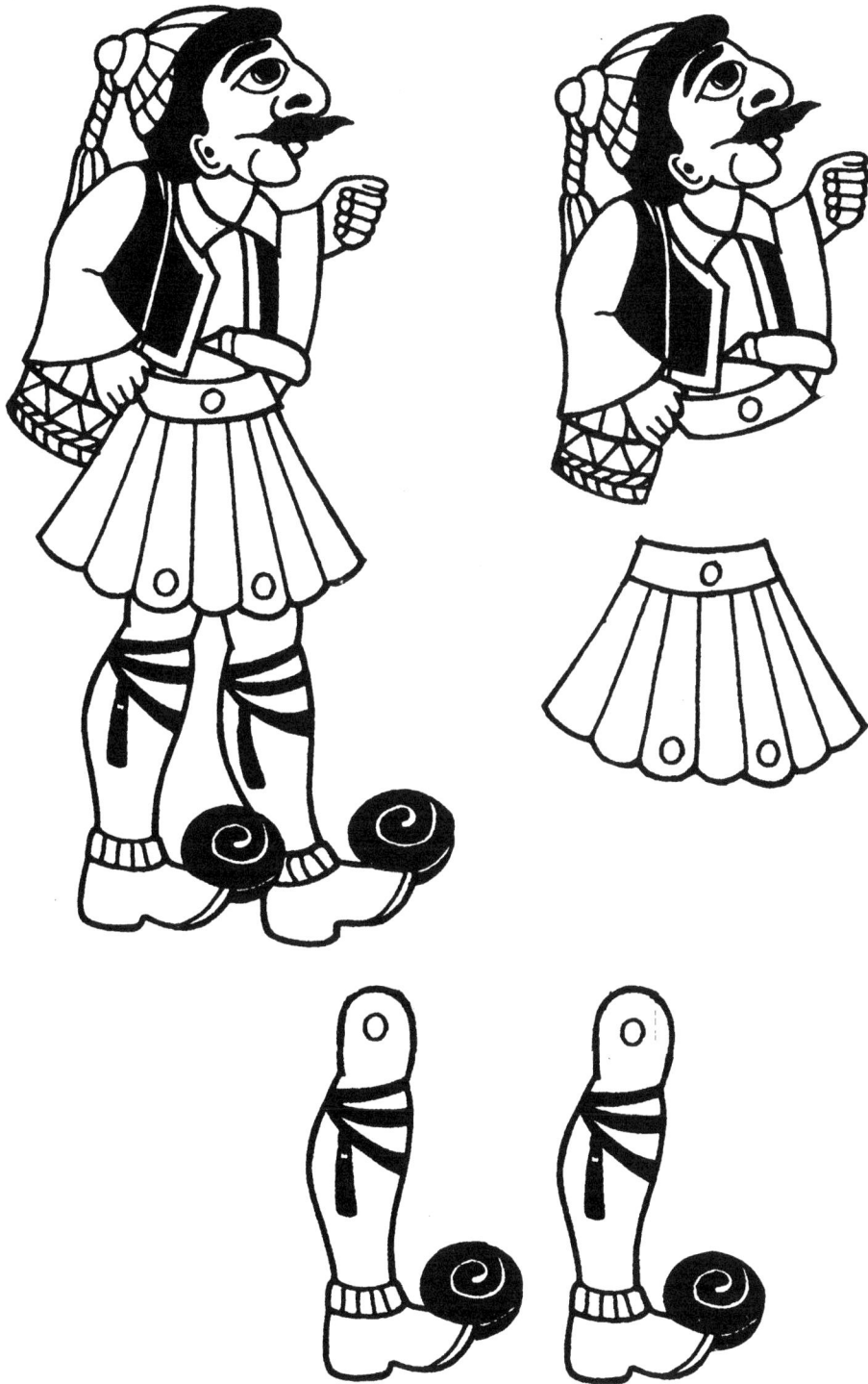

Attach the rod with strong tape on the back just below the neck. The paper fastener at the waist and skirt hem will allow flexibility.

Worksheet 6.4
Scenario between Karaghiozis and Baba Yiorgos

Imagine a meeting between uncle and nephew after Karaghiozis has got into yet another scrape (what might the scrape be?). Create and then script a scene between them. Either read the lines yourself as you move the puppet or invite others to read the lines as you move the puppets.

The Play

Title: _____

_____

_____

_____

_____

_____

_____

_____

_____

_____

_____

You can continue your play on the back of this sheet.

Worksheet 6.5
Greek Shadow Puppets – Morfonios

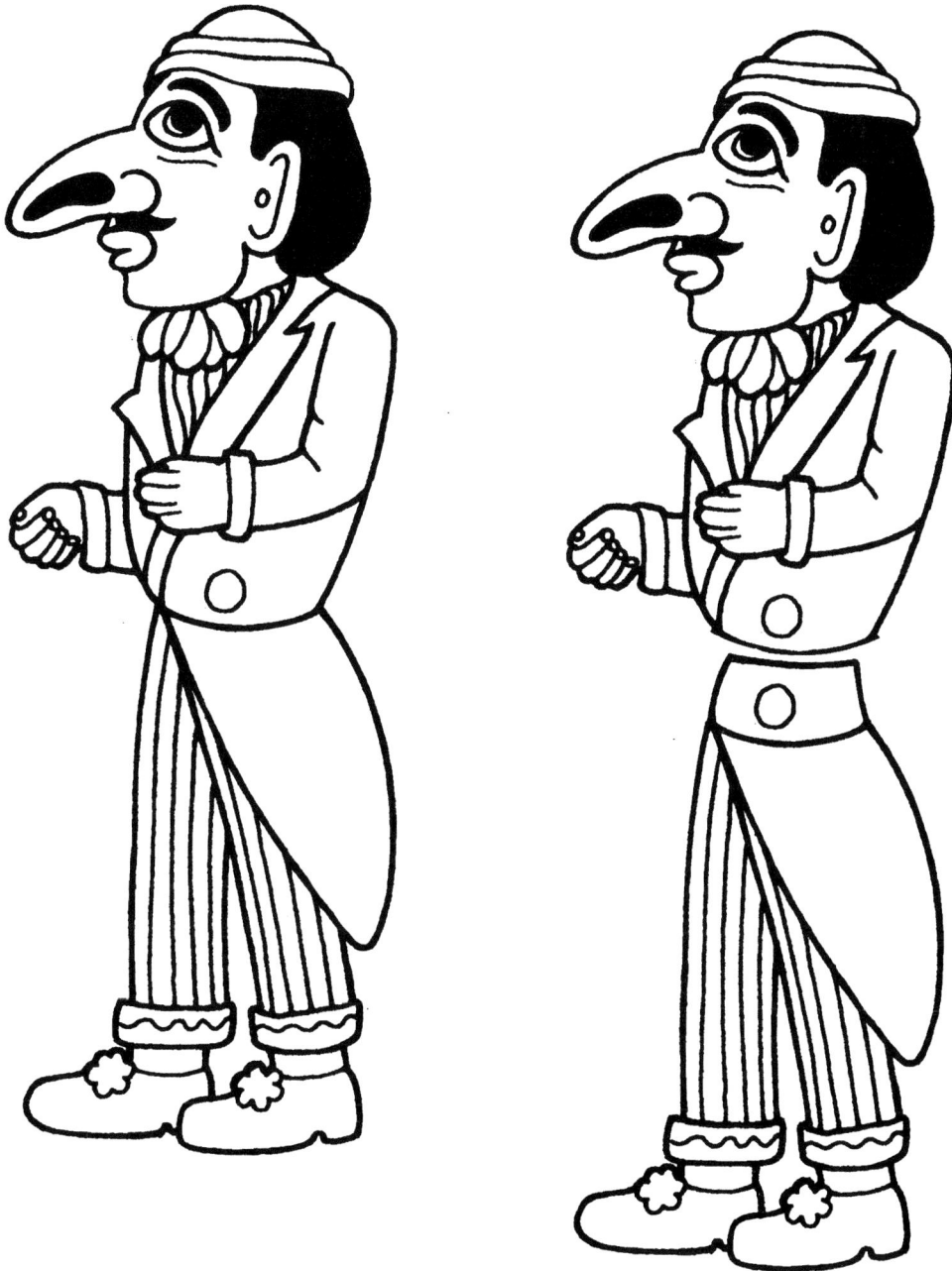

Attach the rod with strong tape on the back just below the neck. The paper fastener at the waist will allow flexibility.

Worksheet 6.5
Greek Shadow Puppets – Morfonios

Side 2

Think about this very definite character and see if you can think up some lines for him to say. Maybe choose some choice lines to indicate his conceit, 'I am better than you', 'I am so handsome that everyone is envious of me'…

Group members or the facilitator can create a speech that Morfonios might say to himself.

_____

_____

_____

_____

_____

_____

_____

_____

_____

_____

_____

_____

_____

You can continue your speech on the back of this sheet.

Worksheet 6.6
Greek Shadow Puppets –
Sir Dionysios

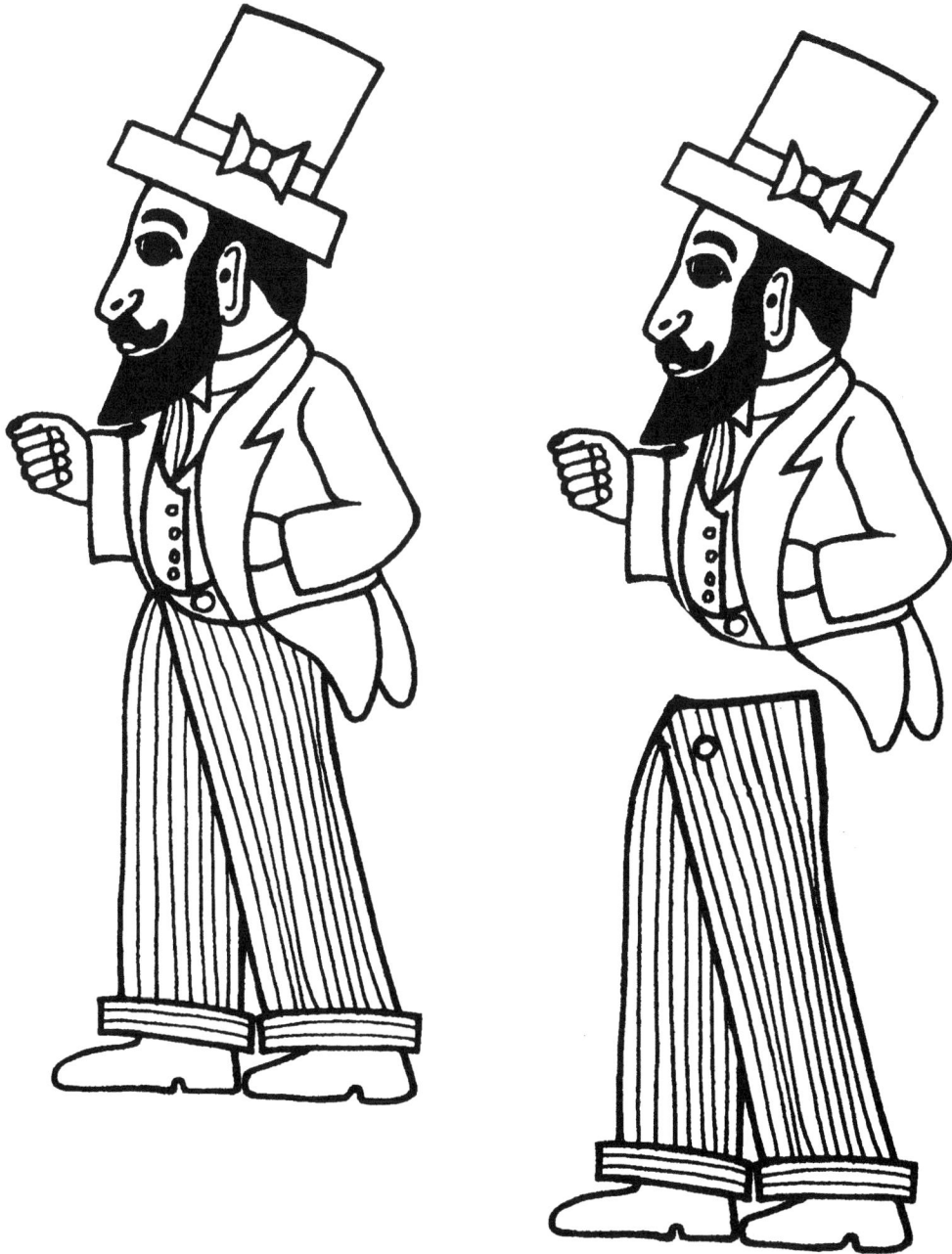

Attach the rod with strong tape on the back just below the neck. The paper fastener at the waist will allow flexibility.

CHAPTER 7

Puppets on Poles

Larger than Life

WHEN I WENT INTO MY HARDWARE SHOP and asked for a dozen broomsticks I received some very funny looks! And of course this is most people's first association with broomsticks; they belong to witches and are ridden through the night with black cats perched on the back of them.

In Chapter 5 we played with the idea of puppets being created out of brooms and mops – with domestic objects that we can find in our houses and workplaces. In many ways the mops are ideal because they already have hair! However, there is less flexibility when creating individual characters from mops and brooms. To do this, we need to make the puppet from scratch.

Let's start with the broomstick – wooden broomsticks that are rounded and smooth and have one end curved and the other end flat. Although there is a push towards plastic sticks, the wooden ones are still available in garden centres and hardware stores. Check them first for splinters and make sure that the floor of your working room will allow some pounding (and the people next door will not be put off by noise!).

Rhythms

Let each person in the group have one broomstick. Stand in a circle and hold the stick upright, with the flat end towards the floor. Use the sticks to beat out a rhythm. Try a simple rhythm to start with, beating 1 – 2, 1 – 2. Be patient; let the group gradually coordinate together. Vary the rhythm for example: beats that are slow, quick, quick, slow; slow, quick, quick, slow. Encourage people to create their own rhythms with partners or in small groups and then share them with the whole group.

Orchestrate the sounds so that people beat louder and more intensely, then quieter and less intense. Encourage individual members of the group to 'conduct' the others.

This rhythm work can gradually develop into more complex patterns, with one group making a slower rhythm and another group making a faster rhythm.

Rhythm work helps people to coordinate sound and movement and to cooperate together. Many people with special needs have difficulties with rhythms and find it hard to establish their own personal rhythm. I have used the broomstick rhythms with teenagers with behavioural difficulties who are reported as being 'out of control'; this also can be considered 'out of rhythm'. People standing, or those in chairs can easily hold the large sticks. For young children the broomsticks can be sawn in half or else use a dowel rod.

Broomstick and Dowel Rod Games

- Stand in a circle and pass one stick round the circle.
- Pass it round the circle and each person passes it hand to hand before passing it on.
- Increase the group's concentration by having more than one stick going round the circle.
- Complex coordination: each person has a stick and passes it round. They will be passing it with one hand and receiving a new stick with their second hand; transferring it to their first hand; then passing on and receiving. Try this out first with friends so that you can give clear instructions! Or you can tell the group the idea and see if they can work it out.
- Left-handed people will be very pleased when the sticks go round the other way and right-handed people will really test their coordination!

Improvisation

Let each person have a piece of dowel rod – roughly 46 cm (18 inches) is ideal:

- Everyone uses it as something sporty (a tennis racquet, golf club and so on).
- Everyone uses the stick as a musical instrument.
- Let members of the group suggest other imaginative ideas (always bearing in mind health and safety issues).
- Suggest that people create something much smaller with it, for example a matchstick.
- Repeat the idea with something much larger, for example a lamp post.
- Let members of the group also suggest ideas.
- In pairs or small groups, invite people to create a scene where the stick(s) are used – but not as sticks or weapons.
- Small groups can create mystery stories where the stick is a vital clue.

This early stick work is important to foster the imagination and encourage people to look at all sorts of possibilities with their sticks, before moving specifically into puppets.

The Puppets

Simple Broomstick Puppet

The simplest way of creating a broomstick puppet would be to follow the instructions in Chapter 5 and attach a painted paper plate to a broomstick. This looks decidedly odd, as if we have a tiny head on a large body. If you want to work with paper plates to make a larger head then construct it as follows:

Paper plate puppet
Use one paper plate as the centre and staple five or six plates round the edge in order to create a very large head.

You will need: paper plates, staples, scissors, coloured paper, crêpe or tissue paper, fabric scraps, masking tape, cotton wool, string or straw.

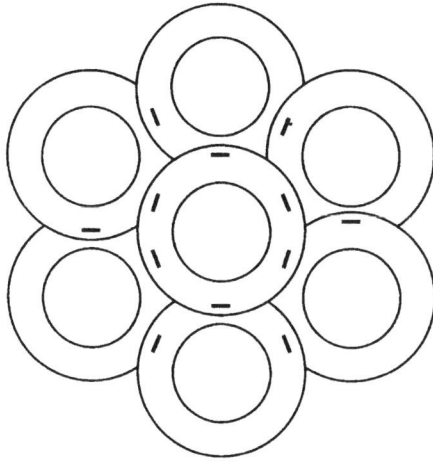

You can also cut the plates in half and staple them to create other interesting shapes.

Once you have the large head, then decide what character you want to create through the addition of painted features: you may wish to stick on eyebrows or mould cheeks and nose with masking tape, or stick on cotton wool; hair made from wool or string or straw can be glued or stapled; you may wish to add some streamers of tissue or crêpe paper.

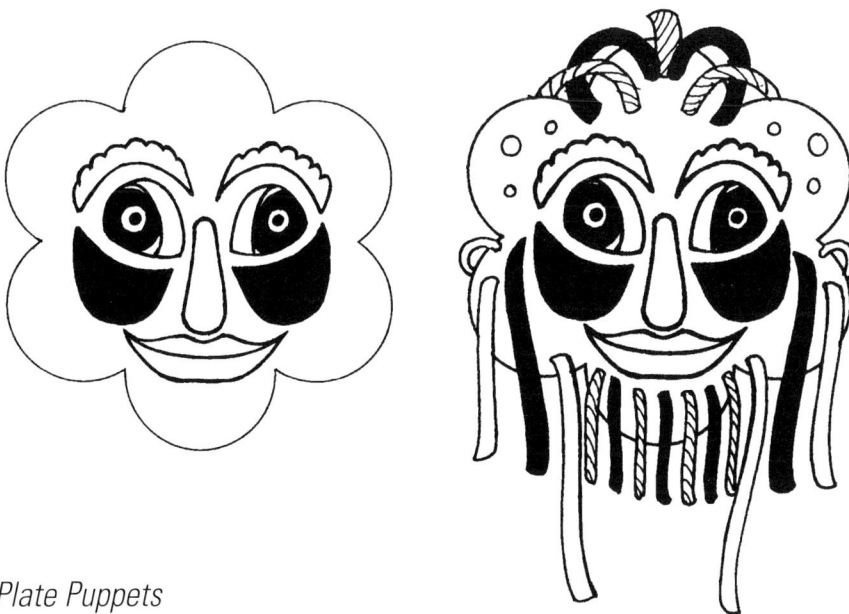

Paper Plate Puppets

When everyone has created their large head, make sure that all the additions are securely fastened, then attach the head to the stick either with masking or duct tape, or with a hinge or loop made of card. It is likely that the sticks will be used again; otherwise you can use wood glue.

Playing with the puppets

- Everyone in the group can introduce their puppet to everyone else: either sitting in a circle or by moving around the room (remember to speak in the first person *as if* you are the puppet).
- The introduction can be very simple: name and where I come from. Or more complex: a little about myself.
- Other members of the group can ask questions (sensible) to help the person elaborate on the character.
- People can decide which puppets can come together in a small group in order to create a story.
- Create stories in small groups: they may be existing stories or ones that the individuals and groups create about their puppets.
- Share the stories in the group.
- Progress beyond the stories in order to create a puppet drama. There are more ideas towards the end of this chapter about 'setting the scene'.

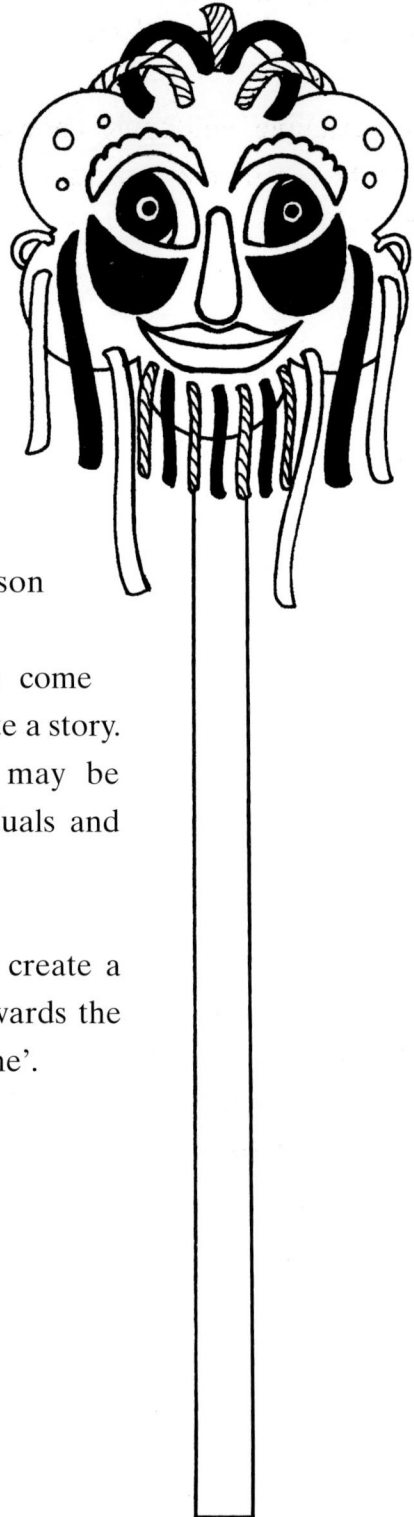

Using Fairy Stories and Myths

You can also use the above technique to re-create the characters from an existing story and then 'script' a puppet play to share either with others or for the group themselves.

For example, you could choose characters from Little Red Riding Hood (Mother, Father/Woodcutter, Grandmother, Wolf – you might want some trees for the wood) or Hansel and Gretel (Father, Stepmother, Boy and Girl, Witch, Bluebird) and tell the stories through the puppets.

Note that both stories have a journey into the woods where dangerous things can happen. If you decide to create the trees using puppets, make sure that everyone has a turn at people puppets and does not have to 'just be a tree'. Although when I created Little Red Riding Hood, the trees were interactive and commented on what was happening like a chorus. They also made lots of sounds and at times the wind whistled through them. (The text for this appears at the end of this chapter in the story sheets.)

Larger-than-life Puppets

Using the broomstick principle of the simple puppets, we are now going to construct a full character with our stick. These characters literally become like large people; through them you can create many different stories and presentations. They can be used for exploring dreams and nightmares and expressing people's feelings. The important thing is that they are being expressed *through* the puppet, which gives additional security if people are feeling vulnerable.

Creating the Puppet

You will need: newspaper, tissue paper, paints, masking tape, thin cloth (optional), glue.

The head Create a head about the size of a football, or a little smaller out of scrunched up newspaper secured with masking tape. Sculpt the features with additional paper and masking tape and paint it in your chosen face colour. Allow it to dry. If you want a smooth finish to the head, then cover it in a layer of thin cloth (beware of it looking like a misshapen Guy Fawkes – unless that is your intention) and then decide how you will create the features. You can also use a layer of tissue paper. Tissue paper and white glue are very good for sculpting features and building up layers such as cheeks or frown lines. Allow the character of the head to emerge and decide what extras you need. For example does your puppet need a hat or cap? What sort of hair will you create? (It could be painted or stuck on.) Does it wear glasses?

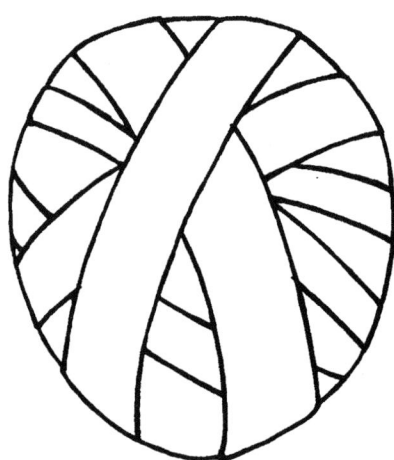

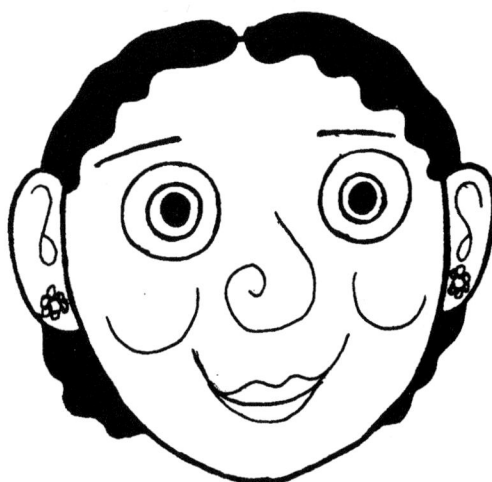

Before you stick the head onto the stick you have to make a decision about the shoulders. If you want shoulders then you need to attach a cross piece of dowel rod which can be firmly stuck with duct tape. Then you can drape your puppet with a shawl or cape, a shirt or a toga. You can play with materials and see what fits your puppet character. Be careful not to make it too complex or too heavy, as this will impede your movement.

If you just want to drape your puppet without shoulders, then create a collar by winding a couple of layers of card, stuck with duct tape, so that any materials you use as drapes do not slip down the smooth wood of the broomstick. You may want to add ribbons or a scarf or a cravat. Maybe your puppet is a mystical character and you can add streamers or wings or a train; think of different head-dresses using various fabrics.

Bore a large hole into the base of the puppet head and push in the broomstick; if the sticks have to be used again, secure it with duct tape, otherwise, use wood glue. Nothing is more frustrating than when a puppet head or the clothes start to turn involuntarily, unless of course you are creating a high comedy show!

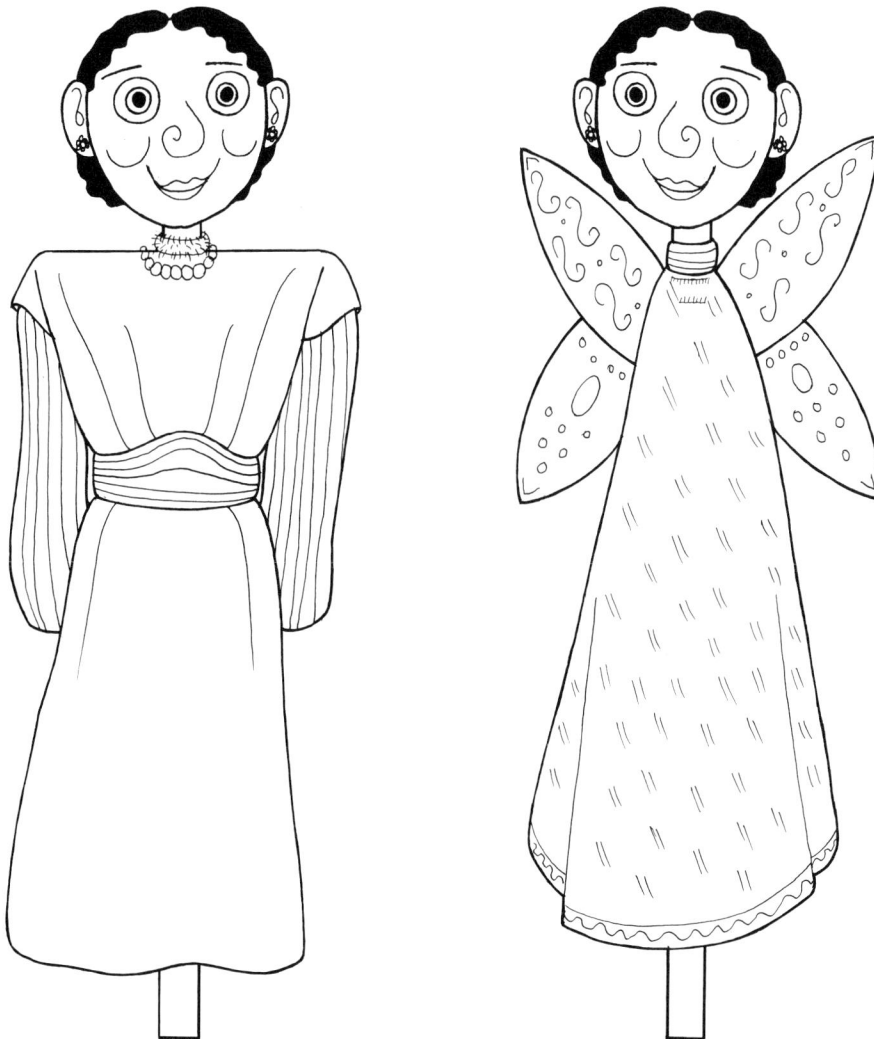

Your large broomstick puppet is now ready for playing and can be developed in many ways. You can use similar warm-up exercises as described for the simple stick puppets, Chapter 5, page 69. However because this puppet has more props and clothes, you will need more time to practise moving with it and feeling confident with its balance. Practise the voice that this puppet has, and think about the details of its character.

Creating the Character

- Write down the name of the character and its details: where it lives, what age – just basic information.
- Write down the feelings that this puppet has and its different qualities: for example the puppet may be shy and timid, or perhaps it is a bit loud and overbearing; it may be feeling sad or angry, and so on.
- What does this character want from life: Dreams? Ambitions? Longings? Fears?
- Write a story about this character in the first person: My name is … and … Create as much detail as you can.
- Free-write about the character in the first person and put in as much information as possible as 'you': who you are close to; who you dislike (from the characters of the story you are creating in the group or from the individual story you have written); what do you need?
- All these techniques are ways for us to get into our characters (whether in puppetry or drama), and will help us create a multi-dimensional puppet that can become very authentic.
- If you are following a particular story then look at the story sheets and use a similar method for creating a puppet performance.

Scenery

It is often helpful to change the environment for puppets and drama, especially when we are working in a setting that conveys other messages. Sometimes it is difficult to play in a classroom that has rows of desks, or in a sports hall that seems overlarge for creative work. I try to keep a supply of large cloths that can camouflage desks and tables; chairs can become props or creatures (they do have four legs!) with added clothes or extensions. For example, a mask can be tied to a chair that is draped with cloth in order to create another character, or even a crowd of characters. An animal head or tail can be added to a chair to transform it. I am sure the group will have lots of ideas once they have been given permission!

Using sticks, rods, cardboard cut-outs and paper plates, you can also create scenery. You can have suns and moons, flowers and trees, outlines of horizons or houses.

Making a Sunflower

Use a large paper plate as a base and cut out golden yellow petals from tissue paper that extend just beyond the edge of the plate. Cut a dark brown piece of tissue to place in the middle and use a felt pen to create yellow dots on the brown centre. Stick the plate to a dowel rod with duct tape, and you have your flower. I am sure you can think of other flowers that can be created in this way. However, a field of sunflowers looks very exciting!

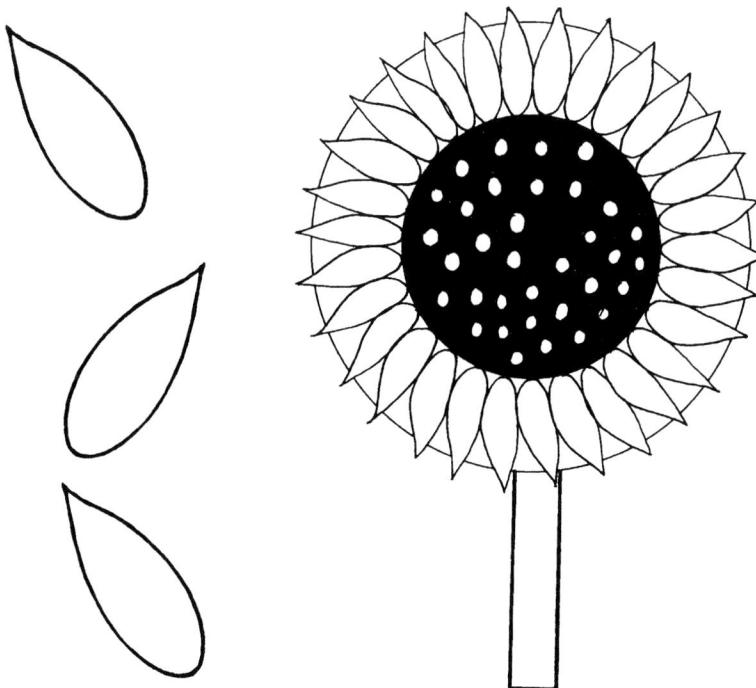

Painting a Backdrop

If you have the facility for hanging a sizeable paper backdrop for the puppet play then use a large roll of paper – you may need to stick together two lengths in order to create enough 'drop'.

Agree with the group what the backdrop should consist of, and perhaps create the picture with a small group of 'stage managers'. Draw outlines and sketches, before attempting the big picture. Keep it simple, with broad sweep images rather than too much finicky detail. For example, you may choose to have a lake as scenery for 'The Children of Lir' story that is described in the worksheets at the end of this chapter.

> **Above all remember that this puppet work is fun, even though it also has a serious purpose. We need to allow ourselves to 'go with the puppet' and we shall find that it takes us to some unexpected places.**

The Story of Red Riding Hood

This is a story for using with the simple broomstick puppets. See Worksheet 7.1 at the end of the chapter for help in staging the puppet show.

Narrator
Many years ago there lives a young girl with her mother and father in a house at the edge of a wood. One birthday she is given a beautiful red cape with a hood and from then on she is called Red Riding Hood.

One day her mother says to her:

Scene One
'Red Riding Hood, you have not seen your grandmother for such a long time – I think I will send you with a basket of food to see how

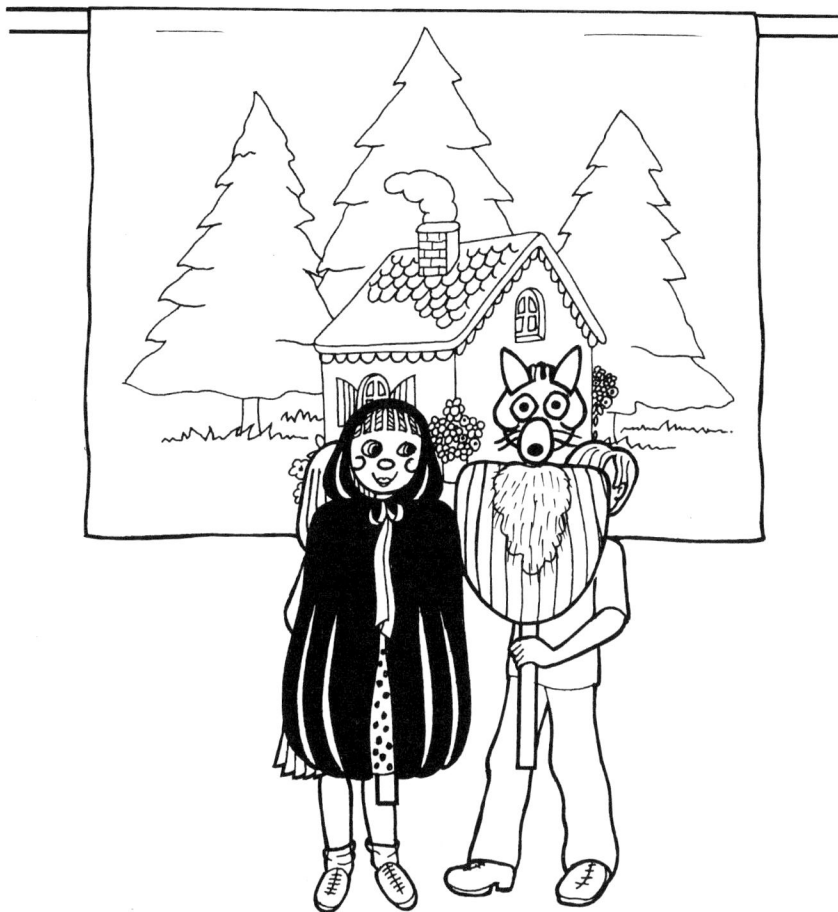

she is,' and she packs some fruit cake and fresh bread and some apples into a basket and covers it with a clean tea towel.

Red Riding Hood puts on her cloak, takes the basket and waves to her mother, 'Goodbye mother, I will be back before sundown,' and her mother stands at the door until she is out of sight, along the little path into the woods.

Scene Two

The wood is wonderful, with all sorts of plants and flowers and a little stream where she sits and has a rest. (The wind is rustling in the leaves and whispering her name.) Walking makes her quite hot! She decides to pick some flowers for her grandmother before continuing her journey. A few moments later a wolf appears, gives her a big smile, and says:

'Good morning little girl! And where are you going on this lovely day?'

(Background noise of trees whispering: 'Red Riding Hood take care – do not trust the wolf – do not trust him.')

'I am going through the wood to visit my grandmother and give her some home-made food,' she says.

'What a good little girl you are; let's have a race – you take this path and I will take that path and we will see who gets there first!' said the wily wolf. And he sets off on the shorter route so he can get there first, and Red Riding Hood walks quickly along the other path.

(And the trees are still whispering to her, but more urgently: 'Don't go there, it is dangerous, don't go there it is dangerous.')

Scene Three
Red Riding Hood arrives at her grandmother's cottage and knocks on the door and her grandmother calls out 'Come in, come in.' She goes inside and upstairs where her grandmother is in bed.

She says, 'Oh Grandma, what big eyes you have.' 'All the better to see you with,' says the wolf who has eaten the grandmother. 'What big ears you have.' 'All the better to hear you with.' 'What big teeth you have.' And the wolf springs out of the bed as he snarls, 'All the better to eat you with!'

Red Riding Hood screams and runs down the stairs, and her father, the woodcutter nearby, hears her and rushes to the house. He fells the wolf with a single blow of his axe and the grandmother climbs out. Red Riding Hood helps her father to secure the house and lay out the lovely food on the table. They all sit down to tea, sandwiches and cake and grandmother is delighted to see her granddaughter again.

Staging the Puppet Play of 'Red Riding Hood'

Text You could use and adapt the story text in this chapter, but you may decide to write your own; experiment with your ideas and decide how much is said by the characters and how much by the narrator.

The puppet Instructions for making the puppets can be found in Worksheet 7.1 at the end of the chapter.

Scenery You may decide to have a painted backdrop with Red Riding Hood's house, and the outline of the wood and a path leading into it. You may decide to create outlines of the different scenes in the landscape. Cut out on card and paint: trees, stream, clumps of flowers, grandmother's cottage, for example and stick onto dowel rods.

Sound effects The story text on pages 114–116 also has ideas for sound effects and whispering voices. Adapt it how you wish, or play with more ideas.

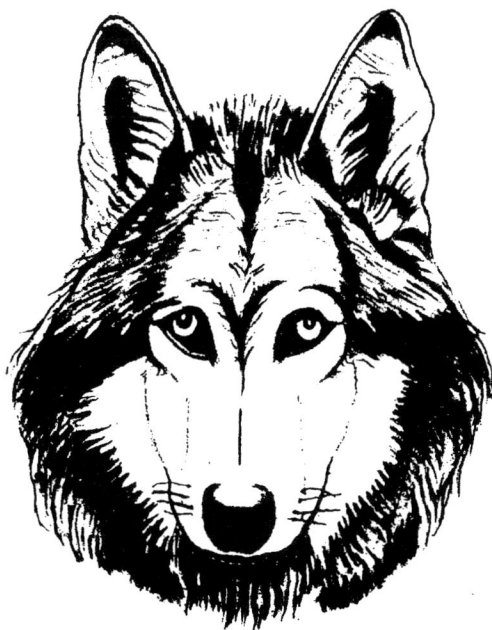

Extra scenes You could add an extra scene where the wolf arrives at the grandmother's house and eats her up; you would then need to make an extra puppet of the grandmother.

Variations Try writing the story of Red Riding Hood from the wolf's point of view. I gave this as a challenge to some young people and the following are some of their ideas:

'I didn't want to eat her grandmother – but she stole and ate my sandwiches!'

'Grandmothers don't taste nice – I would have preferred a pork chop!'

'Why do they exaggerate what happened! She shouldn't have been let into the woods on her own anyway – I just taught her a lesson to be more careful in future – no-one really died.'

The Children of Lir – a Traditional Irish Tale

The Children of Lir is sometimes known as 'The Second Sorrow of Irish Storytelling' and is an ancient story from Celtic times. Worksheets 7.2 and 7.3 offer guidelines on how to create the puppets. There are some extra characters in the story and it is for you to decide whether the narrator will describe them or whether you want more puppets.

The story is a condensed version of 'The Children of Lir'; it has been written about extensively (Daly, 2006; Scott, 2005). The central theme of sorcery and transformation occurs in many cultures and countries, for example, 'The Odyssey', 'The Laidley Worm', and 'The Six Swans'. This story is about loss and grieving and allows us to experience our own feelings of loss while keeping them within a structure and resolution.

The Story

In ancient times, when King Lir of the White Field, who was also known as Lord of the Sea, discovered that he was not to have the head kingship, he went home without giving allegiance to King Dearg, the new head king. The other kings were angry and wanted to pursue Lir, but King Dearg advised them to act in a gentler way: 'I will offer him one of my foster daughters in marriage and he will be bound to us through kinship.'

And so it was that Lir chose the eldest daughter, Ove, and they were married and returned to the White Field. In time Ove gave birth to twins: a son and a daughter, who were named Aod and Fingula. Lir and Ove were overjoyed, and their children were cared for and loved, and soon blossomed. Ove gave birth to twins again, two boys named Fiachra and Conn. However, Ove died giving birth to them and Lir was in despair. It was only his great love for his four children that stopped him from dying of grief.

King Dearg saw the misery of Lir and sent him a message to console him: 'It grieves me too that I have lost a daughter and you a wonderful wife; let us strengthen our friendship and I will give you Ove's sister, Oifa, for your new wife.'

So Oifa married Lir and helped to care for her sister's children and all seemed to be well. However, Oifa began to be jealous of the children and the special place that they held in their father's affection. Soon her jealousy turned to hatred and she decided that things must change in order for Lir to love her just for herself.

One day she decided to take the four children with her in her chariot. Fingula did not want to go as she had a terrible dream that had warned her about Oifa. She was unable to resist her stepmother, and the four of them were taken to the Lake of the Oaks. Oife commanded the villagers there to kill the children but they refused. She became angry and raised her own sword but could not bring herself to cause their deaths. So she drove her chariot into the lake and then put a spell on the children from her ancient art of sorcery. The four children turned into four perfect and beautiful swans, and she sang:

'Leave your father now and live with the birds – your home is now on the waves and the wind.'

Fingula, who had had the prophetic dream sang:

'Now as swans we will find our home with the birds, but our thoughts will travel home to our father. Tell us how long we have to stay as swans, subject to the elements.'

Oifa replied:
'When a man from the north will marry a woman from the south – then shall you be free – you will wander across lakes and seas for nine hundred years – you will keep your children's voices and your songs shall be beautiful.'

Oifa was already beginning to regret what she had done but she could not reverse the spell. She got into her chariot and rode to the castle of King Dearg, where she was asked, 'Where are Lir's children?'

Oifa replied that Lir would not trust his children to Dearg. Dearg sensed that something was very wrong and sent a messenger to Lir to fetch the children. Lir replied that they had already been sent with Oifa, and then he suddenly realised that something terrible had happened. He sank into a melancholy and went to seek his children. He journeyed to the lake and the swans saw him coming and when he arrived they sang for him. They sang the story of what had happened and how they must stay as swans for nine hundred years.

Their father and his people cried out with grief and King Dearg punished Oifa by turning her into a demon of the wind. The swan

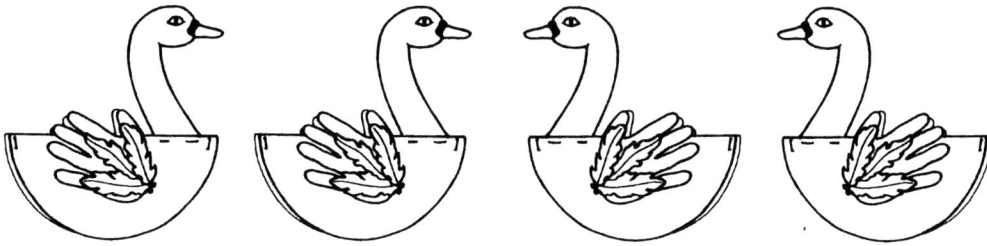

children delighted all the tribes who listened to them singing their magical and sweet songs.

The time came when the storms drove them away from their lake and they flew to a most inhospitable place called the Straits of Moyle. It was cold and icy and the swans were unable to sing their beautiful songs. They became separated in the tempests and ended up cold and afraid. Fingula sang to her brothers to find her at the Lake of Derravaragh. She was overjoyed as they approached, wet and miserable, and she placed Fiachra under her right wing and Conn under her left wing to keep them warm. Aod approached and he was dry and Fingula put him under her breast. So all the swan children were re-united, and they sang songs for the King's messengers that they were well.

At about this time a marriage was to take place between a prince of Connaught, called Lairgnen, and Deoch, daughter of the king of Munster. Deoch had heard about the swans and said she would not wed until she owned them and then they could sing sweetly at her wedding.

It was time for the curse to be lifted from the four swans, and they flew over their old home of the White Field and saw that it was desolate and overgrown. They cried with sadness and flew onwards to the Inish Glora, known as the Bird Isle. There was a monk who had been waiting for them and he asked them to trust him and he joined them together with silver chains.

Lairgnen and Deoch went to the Inish Glora and tried to seize the swans that had been put in sanctuary in the church. As soon as Lairgnen touched them, their feathers all fell off them and there was a very old woman and three very old men. Fingula asked that they be buried in the traditional way which was standing up, with Fiachra and Conn on 'either side and Aod before her'. They were blessed by the monk, then died and were buried just as they had requested.

That night the monk had a dream and he saw the souls of the Children of Lir flying towards the heavens as four most beautiful swans.

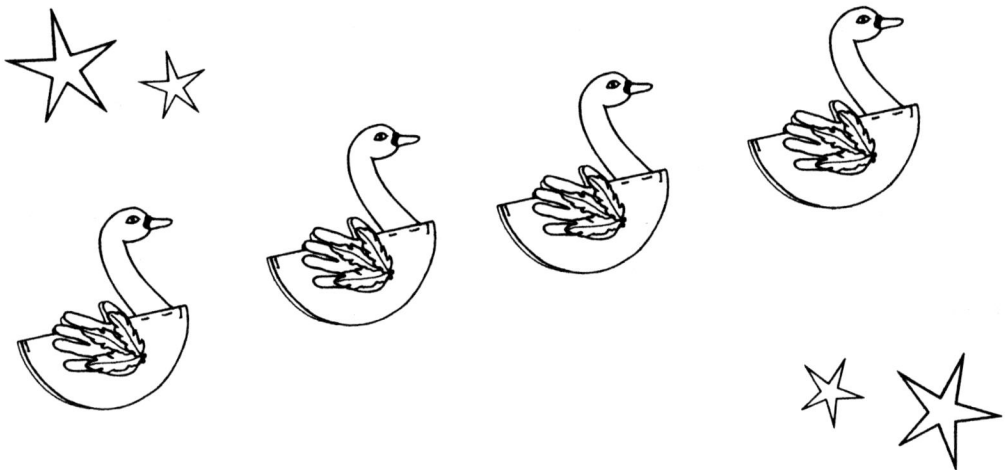

Staging the Puppet Play of The Children of Lir

Text The text is a shortened version of this Irish story, that is sometimes referred to as 'The Second Sorrow of Irish Storytelling'. It has additional scenes at the beginning that include the political situation in ancient Erin (Ireland). This text focuses on the family relationships and the ensuing tragedy of the children.

Scenery You can create a backdrop of the Irish hills and castles, the Lake of Derravaragh, the Straits of Moyle and Inish Glora (later called Bird Isle). You can also create puppet scenery of the different water places, remembering that the Straits of Moyle are very bleak and cold.

Sound effects The children of Lir, once they became swans, retained their human child voices. They also sang very beautifully and plaintively, although in reality swans are mute, and only make a hissing sound. You may want to practise different voices for the characters including the mutterings of the crowd of villagers. Think about other sound effects that could increase the power of this story.

Further research There are many stories that have the theme of humans turning into swans and back again. Think of the story of the ballet 'Swan Lake', and other legends. Find out as many stories as you can and ponder the importance of the swans in this context. What is the historical reason that swans are a protected species in the UK and a third of them owned by the Queen?

Worksheet 7.1
Puppets on Poles — Red Riding Hood

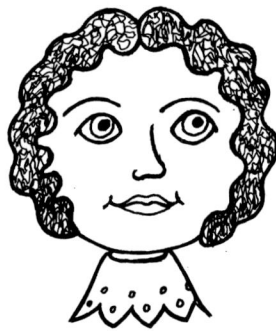

You will need: paper plates, a broomstick for each character, a dowel rod for each tree, paints, PVA glue, masking tape, duct or parcel tape, strong stapler, scissors, scraps of material, wool, tissue paper.

Follow the instructions for the simple broomstick puppet (on pages 106–108), and create the following characters:

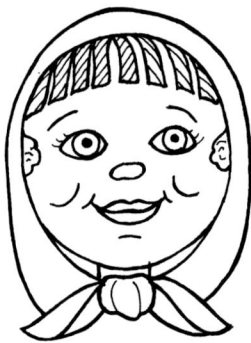

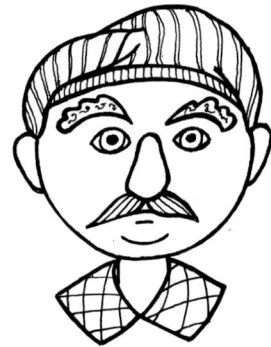

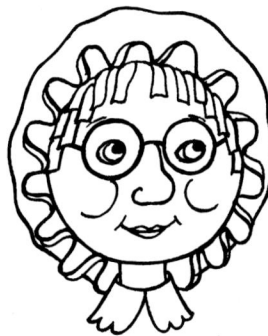

Red Riding Hood	Her mother	Her father, a woodcutter
Mr Wolf	Her grandmother	Mr Wolf as grandmother
Background trees	Grandmother's cottage	

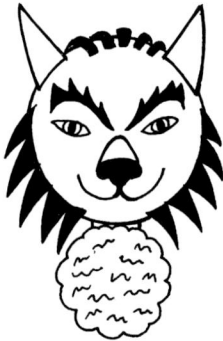

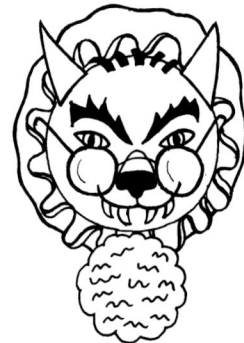

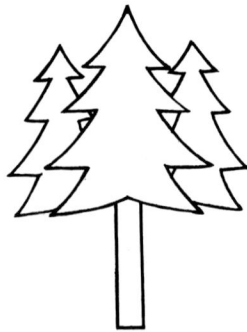

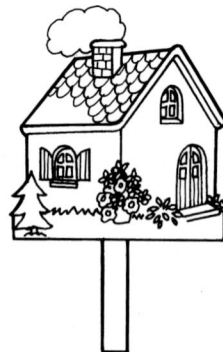

Worksheet 7.2
Puppets for The Children of Lir

To create these puppets you will need: broomsticks and dowel rods, newspapers, masking tape and duct tape, paint, cloths for dressing and draping, head-dresses, hats and crowns.

Characters
King Lir of the White Field
Ove: his wife
His four children: twin son and daughter, Fingula and Aod; twin sons, Fiachra and Conn
Oifa: their stepmother
Dearg: The Head King
Messengers and local people
Four swan heads (to create a swan puppet see Worksheet 7.3)
One monk

Create all the puppets apart from the messengers, local people and swan heads as broom puppets with the newspaper heads. Choose the costumes and head-dresses carefully, remembering that Dearg is more senior than Lir. Ove and Oifa are sisters. Ove is described as a woman of the day, and Oifa as a woman of the night and a sorceress.

Create the messengers and villagers from paper plates or card cut-outs, paint them and stick them onto dowel rods; group members can hold one in each hand.

The four swan heads can be sculpted with newspaper and masking tape, so there is at least 22.5 cms (9 inches) of neck. Use the guide on Worksheet 7.4 to get the swan shape and then paint white with orange beaks and black breathing nostrils. Use dowel rods to extend the neck.

Worksheet 7.3
The Children of Lir –
creating a Swan Puppet

You will need: two 22.5cm (9 inch) paper plates, white construction paper, scissors, a black marker, white craft feathers, stapler and staples, white glue.

1 Fold two paper plates in half. Align them at their folded edges and staple them together at each end.
2 Trace your hands on white paper. Cut the hand shapes out for wings. Glue a wing on each side of the plates. Glue some feathers on the wings.
3 Draw a head with beak and neck, and an eye each side with a pupil in the centre of each eye.
4 Staple the head and neck to the inside of the swan body.
5 Attach to a stick or dowel rod.

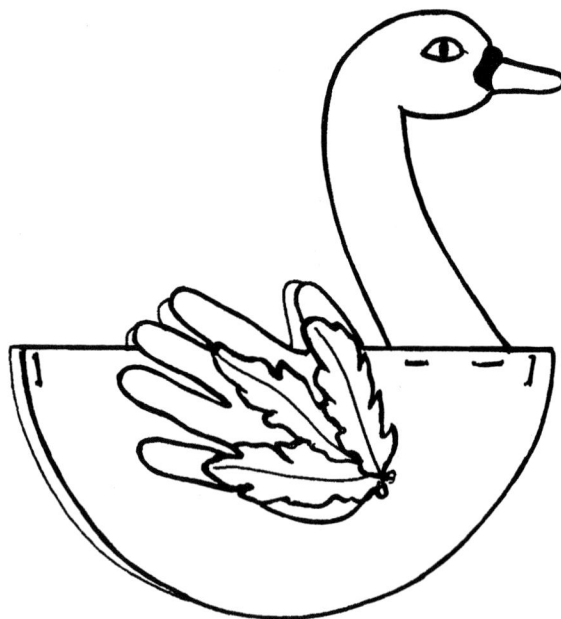

Worksheet 7.4
The Children of Lir – alternative Swan Puppet

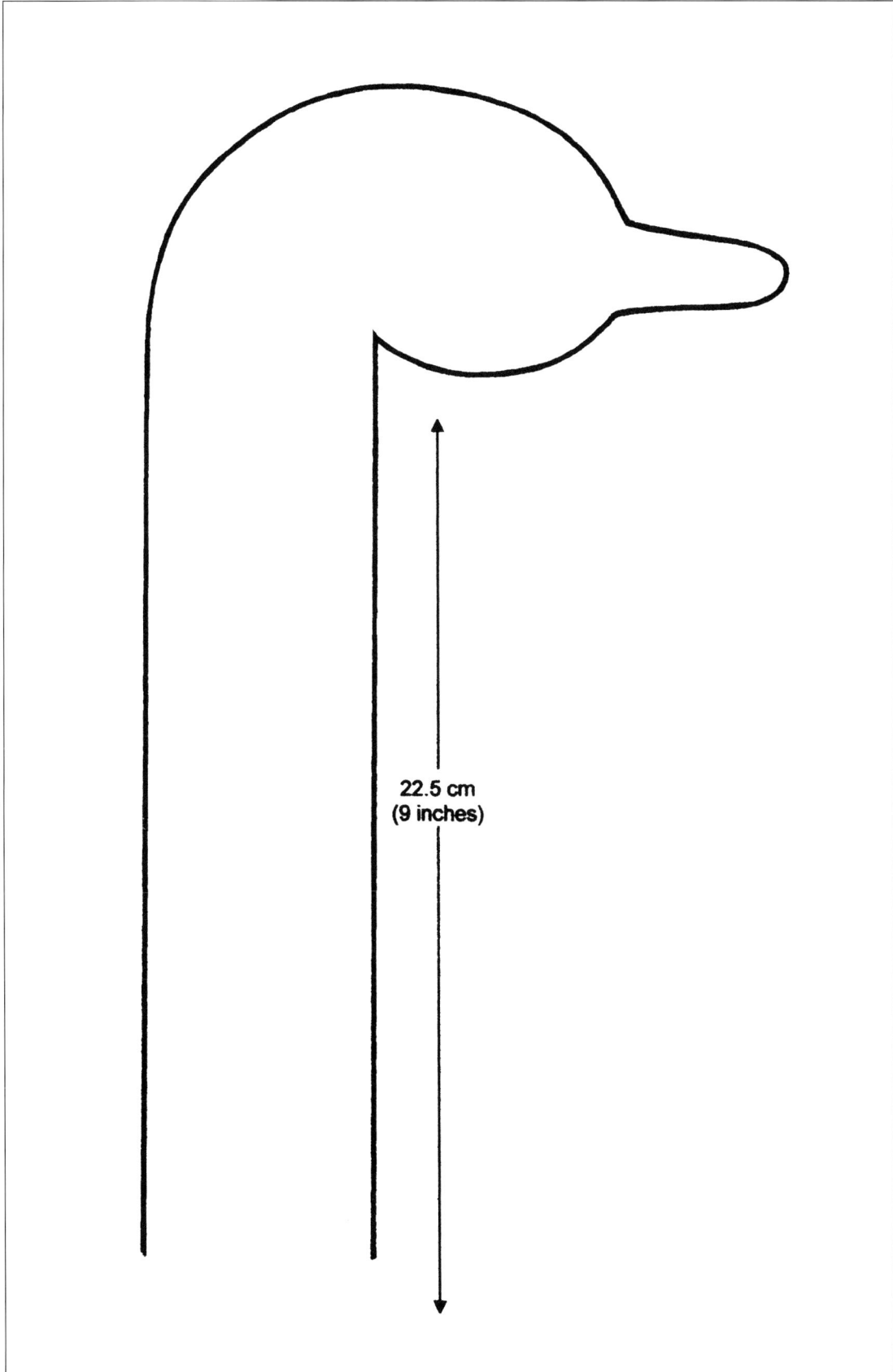

22.5 cm
(9 inches)

CHAPTER 8

Puppets with Mouth

I N THIS CHAPTER YOU WILL FIND BIG-MOUTHED PUPPETS, generational puppets, animal puppets with moving mouths and finger puppets. They have inspired a number of stories by children which are reproduced here.

There are now many puppets available which have mouths that move so that they can 'speak'. Many of them are reminiscent of the puppets used on television shows and at times they can create 'silly voices' rather than encourage the authentic voice of the child. However, if mouth puppets are chosen carefully, puppets that speak can play an important role both in education and therapy. If we use stereotyped puppets then children and adults will often just reproduce the catch phrases and expressions that they have heard through the media, and indeed will perhaps think that is our expectation. However the exception can prove the rule and I have known an adult work with Kermit the frog as a character that he felt he had to play in his life, and was eventually able to go beneath the 'public face' and explore new ways of being for himself.

Big-mouthed Puppets

The largest mouth puppets are also able to move their hand and fingers so a child can use one hand to move the mouth and the other hand to create movements and gestures with a hand. Some children enjoy playing with both hands moving inside the puppet's hands instead of manipulating the mouth. They are big enough to sit on the adult's or child's lap and tell stories or hold a conversation.

I have two of these puppets on my play room shelf. One is dressed in very raggedy clothes, possibly bought from a charity shop, and I call her Rainbow Jane. You will have met this puppet in *Creative Storytelling with Children at Risk* (Jennings, 2004a) when we discussed working with the motif of rainbows. Rainbow Jane is a streetwise character and beloved by children of all ages. She

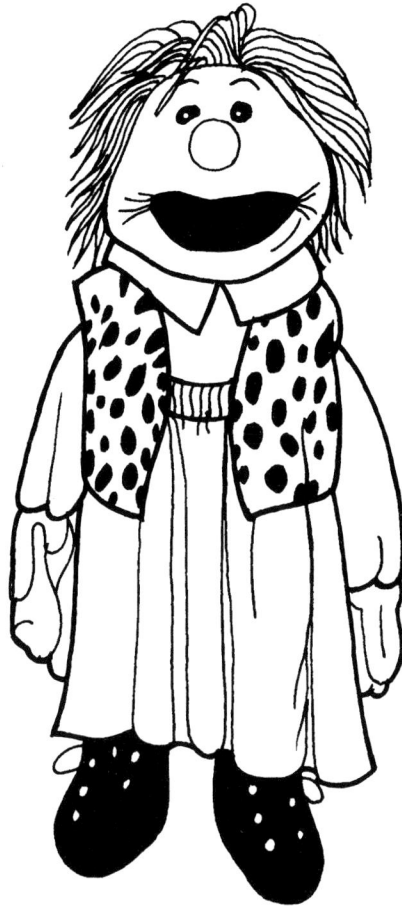

has lived on the street and travelled the road and picked up all sorts of stories. She has been in all sorts of scrapes and survived to tell the tale. Children see her as an ally as well as someone who can give them guidance. She does not take on the role of 'wise person' as that would imply an older character. No, Rainbow Jane is a contemporary and a puppet with which most children can identify. Perhaps we could refer to this approach as 'peer puppetry'!

Rainbow Jane and Football Louie

Rainbow Jane listens to troubles, gives advice from her own experience and generally is able to reflect with a young person on the best way forward. She is also good at interactive storytelling. She has a friend called Football Louie.

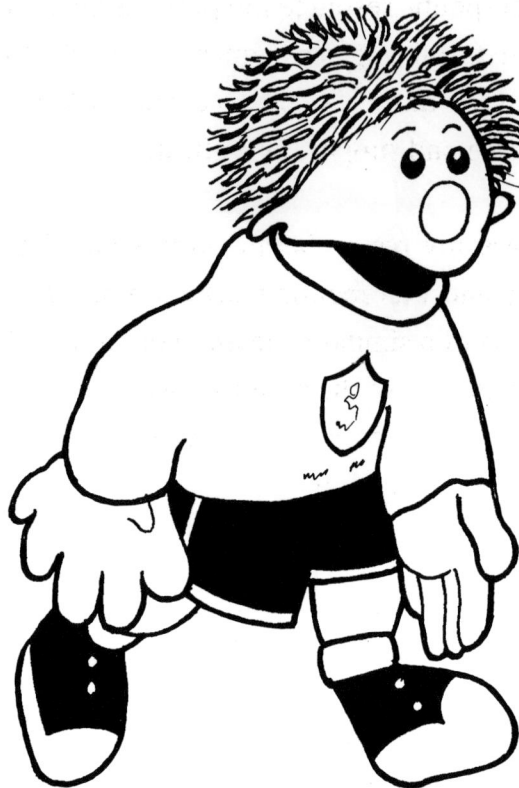

Football Louie is less patient than Rainbow Jane and can speak out of turn! Sometimes Louie needs to ask help from Rainbow Jane to get him out of scrapes. However, he is likeable and loveable and very popular with boys and girls. He does not always get things right and drops things and opens his mouth rather than waiting and listening. None of his social misdemeanours are too extreme, but nevertheless his life would be easier if he could remember some ground rules.

These two large puppets have many uses both in therapy and education. People often want to have both working together and will sometimes want the therapist to have Louie, while they play the more knowledgeable role through Jane. At other times children and adults will want the therapist to have the puppet and for them to ask the questions.

Both puppets are asked to tell stories that include stories about their own lives, 'Have you ever done that...?', as well as stories for new directions and stories for soothing or calming.

As well as being a therapeutic resource the puppets are excellent puppets for use in education and training programmes, especially for learning social skills. Louie can make the mistakes and Jane can invite comments and then encourage skills practice and support and affirm.

These two puppets are my particular favourites and I find they are very flexible for education and therapeutic work with all age groups. However, there are many puppets of a similar style and you may find you prefer other characters. It is important to like the materials we work with and then we will be more authentic in our creativity and expression (please see Useful Addresses for resources for puppets).

Generational Puppets

There are several puppets that represent grandma and grandpa and many that represent children and teenagers, but I am still searching for parent puppets. Although the grandmas and grandpas are all white puppets, they are very popular with all age groups.

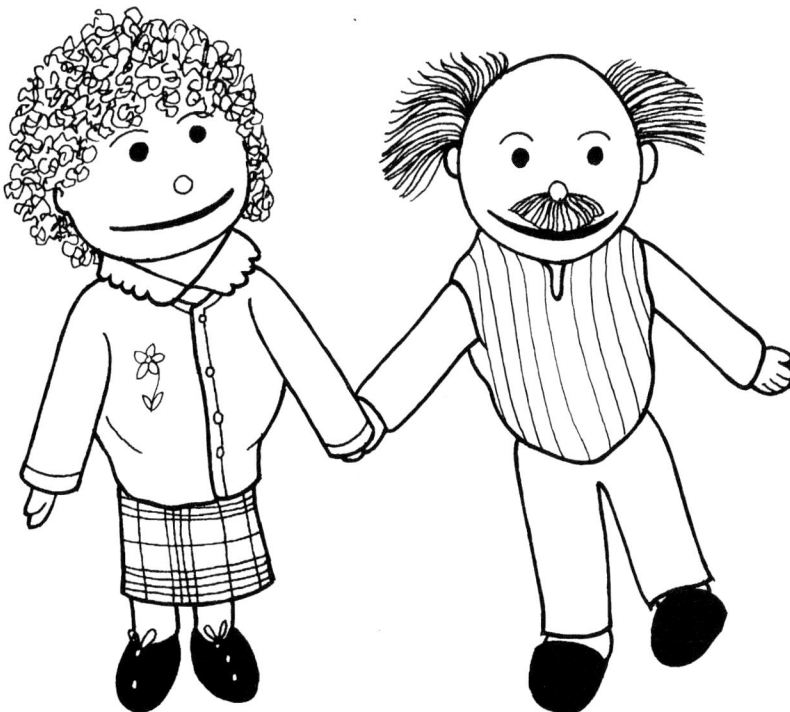

Rather than being media characters, they present another type of stereotype of a safe elderly person who is wise and stable. The grandma, in particular, usually takes on the role of the 'comfortable granny' who is patient and listens. The following is a description of grandmothers by a twelve year old boy:

> *A grandmother is a woman who has no children of her own, and therefore she loves the boys and girls of other people. Grandmothers have nothing to do. They only have to be there. If they take us for a walk they go slowly past beautiful leaves and caterpillars. They never say 'Come along quickly' or 'Hurry up for goodness sake'. They are usually fat but not too fat to tie up our shoe strings. They wear spectacles and sometimes they can take out their teeth. They can answer every question, for instance why dogs hate cats and why God isn't married. When they read to us they do not leave out anything and they do not mind if it is always the same story. Grandmothers are the only grown-ups who always have time. Everyone should try to have a grandmother, especially those who have no television.*

Grandmothers may be good at reading stories and may take their grandchildren on their nature walks. Attitudes towards grandfathers may be more complex, depending on a child's (or an adult's) experience. Some children coming to therapy may use the grandpa puppet to disclose abuse from grandfathers or uncles, or to start to explore what has happened to them. We need to follow the child or adult in their perception of the puppets and what they are trying to tell us through the puppet.

We must be careful not to make assumptions as to how someone will see a puppet. Individuals will project their own images on to a puppet and we need to hear that, or the person may feel, yet again, that they are not listened to or believed.

If disclosure happens out of therapy then we need to acknowledge and not respond with shock or disgust. The individual needs reassurance that they will have some help.

Of course if there is disclosure regarding abuse in our sessions then we need to follow the procedures in place for reporting abuse to the appropriate authorities. Unfortunately, not all schools have procedures for reporting bullying and intimidation, and that is something that perhaps we should request in our work setting.

It is important that there are puppets who can speak about bullying, as well as black and Asian puppets, and puppets that are not 'tough'.

Nevertheless, in the main the grandfather puppet is a supportive and helpful character; sometimes he is a bit short-tempered and impatient. He is the character that Mary developed in her story about the man and the cat. The cat was a white cat sleeve puppet:

Story for a Cat and a Man Puppet
by Mary

Once upon a time there lived a cat called Millie. Millie lived on the road and had no food, so she looked through bins and she always saw a fish so she ate it. When it was night Millie could not go to sleep because the owls hooted. Somewhere in the town a door had been left open. It had been left open because the man who lived in that house had no air. It squeaked and creaked. So the man who lived in that house couldn't go to sleep as well.

So Millie went in the man's home and said, 'Please can you shut that door?' 'No I cannot shut the door.' 'Why?' said Millie. 'Because I won't have any air,' said the man. 'Oh sorry,' said Millie. 'That's all right, thank you,' said the man. 'But please can you shut that door, OK?' said Millie.

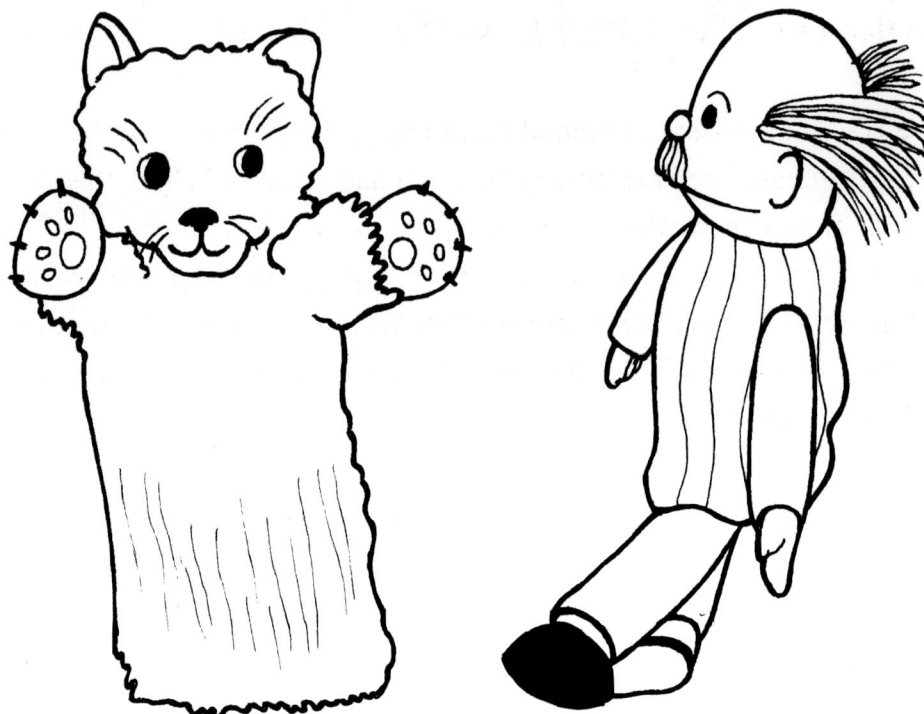

Now everyone could not sleep because the door was squeaking and creaking. Everyone gathered around the man's house talking and chattering, then someone said, 'Put some oil on the door'. 'OK,' said the man. Now Millie was very happy.

Then she went back to her den and when she got to her den she had forgotten something and she did not know what it was. So she went to the man's house and asked him, 'What is so special about tomorrow?' 'It's your birthday,' said the man. 'Oh yes!' said Millie. 'OK, OK now go back to your den,' said the man. 'Why?' said Millie. 'Because you've got a big day tomorrow, OK?' said the man.

And Millie went to her den and she slept until her birthday started. And when she woke up she saw lots of toys and people and she said thank you.

THE END

Animal Puppets with Moving Mouths

There is a huge variety of animal hand puppets that include both domestic and wild animals. They are usually very soft and furry, and children enjoy the fact that they can stroke them. There are some hand puppets that have extended bodies and are called 'sleeve puppets' that are easier to manipulate. They have small mouths that little fingers are able to open and close as if they are talking. Worksheet 8.2 gives instructions for making a simple animal puppet.

The range of puppets means that a child is not limited in their expression, and we need to be careful that we do not impose our own associations with the animals. For example the rat puppets are very popular, especially with boys, who otherwise would think that puppet work is sissy and very uncool! In one-to-one therapy, some children and teenagers would be horrified if they thought their peers knew that they came to 'play' and indeed many parents are at a loss to know why playing can be therapeutic. Adults so often have difficulties in playing and the puppets are often a way through the troughs and sloughs.

Furry puppets can be cuddled like 'soft toys' but they have a little more status, especially when they are wild animals. By far the most popular wild animal in my collection is the sleeve wolf puppet. He has teeth and a large tongue and although very soft and cuddly, he has a tough persona. I do not specify gender but most people think it is a he: however, sometimes stories get told about protective she wolves.

The image of the wolf, although much maligned in the past, (the Christian churches believed that wolves were in league with the devil and sometimes people had to be exorcised from their wolf familiar) is in reality a model for a stable family. Wolves stay together and protect their young against all the odds. Although historically they were slaughtered and wiped out in many countries, they are now a protected species in most countries and there is talk of re-introducing them into Scotland.

The wolf hand puppets developed into a wolf project with pictures and story writing for children and teenagers. The following are examples of the stimulation of the imagination that was provoked by the theme of wolves.

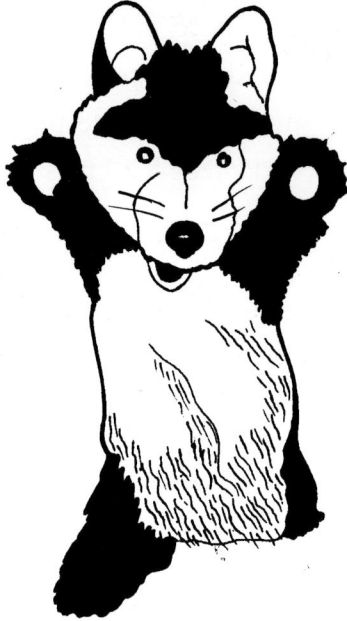

The Fight of Rabbit and Wolf
by Kaia

A long time ago there was a wolf and a rabbit. They were very bad enemies. This is how it started.

The rabbit once bit him because he was the king and he wanted to be the king so they became bad enemies. The next week he gathered up people to fight him [the wolf]. *So the next day when the wolf went down to get something to eat they all jumped on him and they hurt him but the wolf jumped up really high and the rabbit and the other people were scared that he was going to jump on them so all of them ran away.*

But after two weeks he found a sword and a shield and the next day when he came down to get something to eat all of them jumped out on him and hurt him. Then he picked up a chair and pretended to throw it at him and the rabbit thought he was actually going to throw it at him so he ran away again.

He didn't come back and so he was very safe indeed.

And that night he felt luvily.

THE END

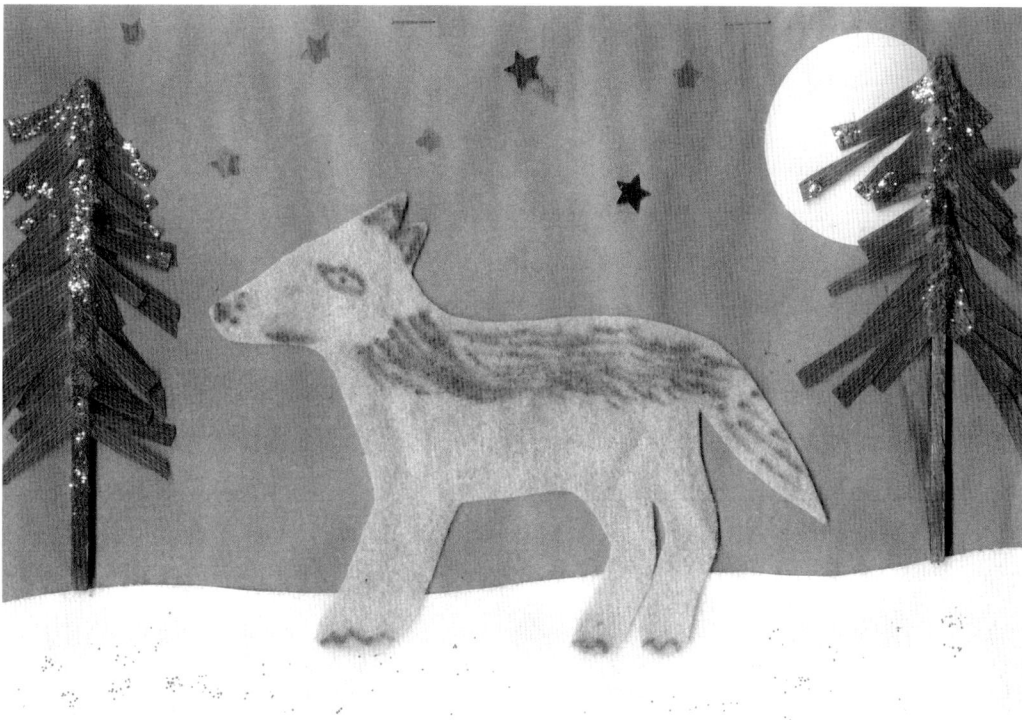

By Sorrel

The Black Wolf
by Alex

In a forest that was as green as grass, stood a wolf moving his light grey and active eyes from side to side, protecting his pack from an attack. This wolf was not like most wolves, he was black and a lot smaller than the rest. As he was looking around he noticed far away in the distance, his old pack's jungle in bright yellow flames.

The sight of the flames churned back his mind to when he was little and when his pack had been hunted down by man 8000 years ago.

Next morning, Scarfish, the Black Wolf alerted the rest of them that they had to move, there were men on the way. When the news spread through the pack there was utter terror. As they were getting ready they heard a shout and Black Wolf ran over to where the sound was coming from. As he rushed over he spotted that behind a bush there was a man. He was lying on the floor, screaming for help. Black Wolf tried to say,

*   'What happened', but all that came out was*

*   'Aooooh', which did not seem to help much so Black Wolf walked towards him, caught hold of his shirt and tugged him back to Base.*

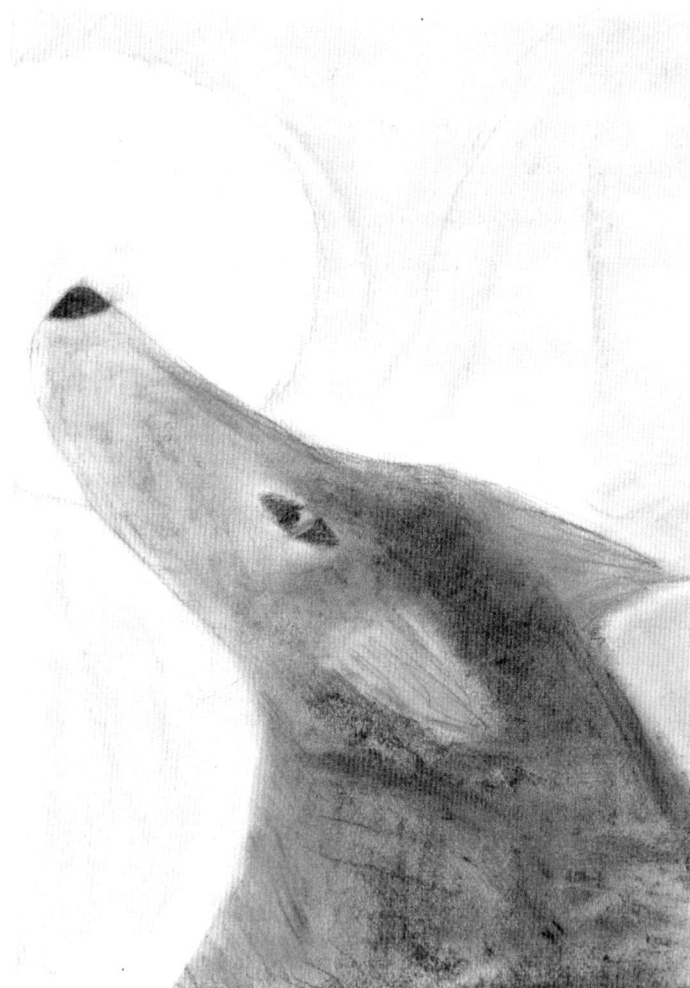

By Laura

'What's this', asked Parrot.

'A person from the hunters', he answered. Everyone gasped. A little pig ran to hide behind his mum.

'We've got to heal him', said Black Wolf. With that he started licking his [the man's] wound with his tongue.

'Why?' asked Parrot, but Black Wolf didn't answer and this seemed to agitate the Parrot. No other Wolf would try to heal a man, even if they had special powers like Black Wolf. He had only been licking for a couple of minutes when the wound disappeared. The man jumped up and looked straight at his ex-scar. He looked back at the Wolf and said,

'Are you magical?' Black Wolf now knew, he could talk to this man, he had healed him.

'In a way, yes, but now I have done you a favour, I would like you to do me a favour', Black Wolf answered. 'Tell your men to stop'. As he spoke, men gathered round and aimed their rifles but the man stood in the way and said

'STOP!' The men put down their rifles and the chief choked.

'What are you doing, gooli?'

'Stopping you from killing these animals, they healed me'. With that they all knelt down in front of Black Wolf and said

'Your wish is my command'.

THE END

The Good Wolf
by Yasmin

You know the story of Little Red Riding Hood. This is my point of view. The wolf of Miss Hood from her point of view. I am the Bad Wolf. It wasn't my fault. I ate her gran I was hungry any way I was aiming for a pork chop. Look this is the hood story, it started like this.

Little red riding hood was running to her granma and I could smell the sandwiches so I followed her. She got to her granma's. she knocked and knocked again. At the end she just went in gave her gran the sandwiches and went down sta[i]rs. So I went up sta[i]rs and ate her! Well she ate the sandwiches that I was going to eat!

I heard Little Red Riding Hood's foot steps so I rummaged in her Granma's wardrobe and found some clothes and put them on. She thought I looked a bit like her Gran but she had put makeup on so she went home and I raided the cupboards and ate everything but the biscuits. I don't like biscuits.

So I went home with a full stomach and still chewing some crisps and a bottle of orange squash in my rite hand.

THE END

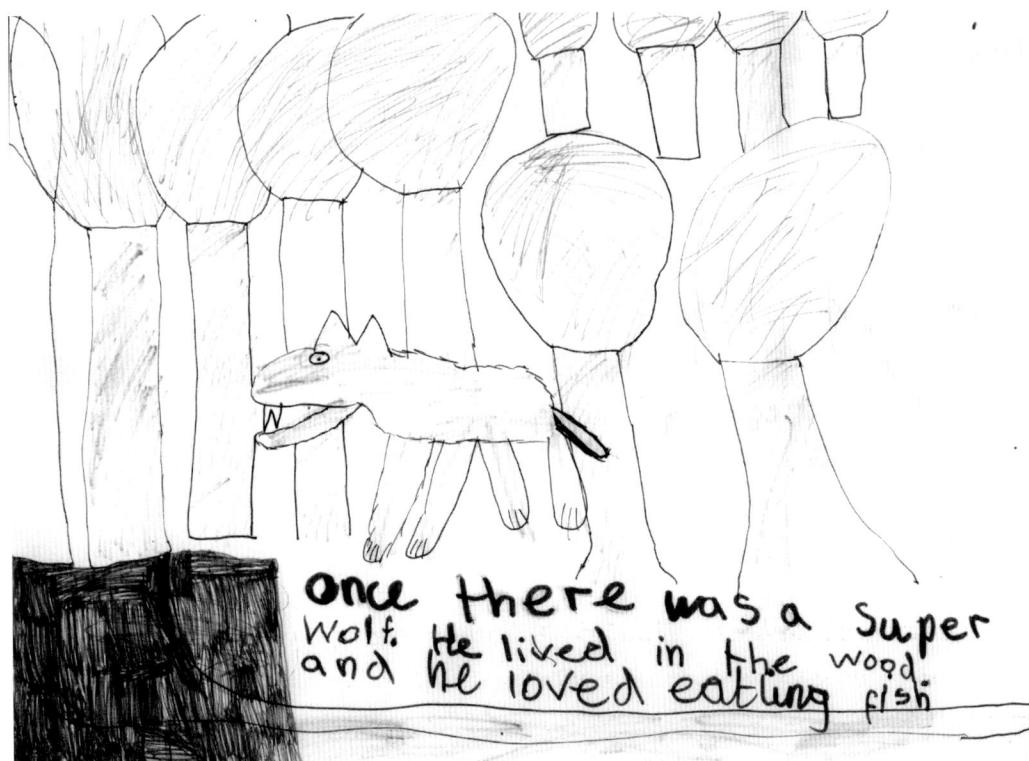

once there was a super wolf. He lived in the wood and he loved eating fish

By Mary

The Dragons of Glastonbury Tor

Glastonbury Tor is a famous hill that stands like a beacon for miles around. They say you can see the Tor for miles and from its top you can see seven counties. There are many tales about the Tor but this one is little known as it could affect the Tor for ever.

Jade and Corin decide they are going for a walk up the Tor – they have been before and it is always a favourite place. They climb and climb and gaze at the sheep grazing peacefully, cropping along the spiral path. As they stand still, Jade nudges her brother, 'We haven't greeted the dragons, you know we must always tell them we are here,' she says, 'Oh yes, let's do it now' and they both lie flat on the ground and put their ears to the ground. Corin mouths to his sister, 'Can you hear them breathing?' 'Yes, like always,' she whispers. They both gently drum on the ground as a way of paying their respects to the dragons.

As they jump up and continue their walk they are aware that a mist is swathing round them, they can just see ahead of them. Jade stumbles, and calls out to Corin, 'We have to stop and go back, we cannot see the top anymore' and they both stop and turn, but the way behind them is completely obscured by the instant Somerset mist, moving and swirling but completely opaque. 'We are lost' wails Corin, and looks as if he is about to cry. 'No we are not,' says Jade forcibly. ' We know just where we are – on the Tor about half way up – we just can't see our way in front or behind – it will change soon.'

They both sat down on the hill side and snuggled up to each other and waited for the mist to move away. 'Tell me the dragon story' says Corin. 'There are so many' laughs Jade, 'Let's tell the tale of the water springs. Keep your hands on the ground and maybe the dragons will hear it through our bodies. Now listen carefully and sit still.'

'Inside the Tor are the sources of two wonderful springs known as white spring and the red spring. These springs have been there since

the beginning of time and they never dry up. That's because they are guarded by the White Dragon and the Red Dragon.'

'We've been to the springs and drunk the water, do you remember?' she says to her brother, and he nods, already absorbed in her story, 'And you can taste the iron in the red spring and the water from the white spring is much milder.'

'The two dragons have been sleeping for thousands of years and the water continues to flow. People come from miles around to drink this water because it has special minerals and many people think it is healing too.

'But now things are changing and many people think that the dragons are on the move. The water is much more difficult to get now, and people think they can control it and then ...'

Before she could say another word, a voice came out of the mist, 'And the people did not learn that the dragons should be listened to until it was too late.' And a tall figure came up to the children, wearing a long black cloak and his white hair flowing down his back. 'But I think you children should go home. Come, I will take you off the Tor. You're good children and you know what is right.'

He strode off and the children followed close and in no time at all they were off the hill and the mists had disappeared. There was their street leading to home and their Mum was standing in the front garden waiting for them and waving. They turned to thank their guide but the street was empty. 'Where can he be?' said Corin, 'Shhh,' said Jade, 'Not a word to Mum, she will think we've been talking to strangers.' 'Was he really there?' said Corin. 'Well, I remember what he said' said Jade, 'Do you?'

'And the people did not learn that dragons should be listened to until it was too late.'

This story can be told through the dragon moving mouth hand puppet as a narrator or you can have several hand puppets. The children can be small moving mouths buddies, and you have the two dragons who can be heard breathing and later moving away if you want to extend the story. You can paint a back drop for the Tor like the children in the pictures below.

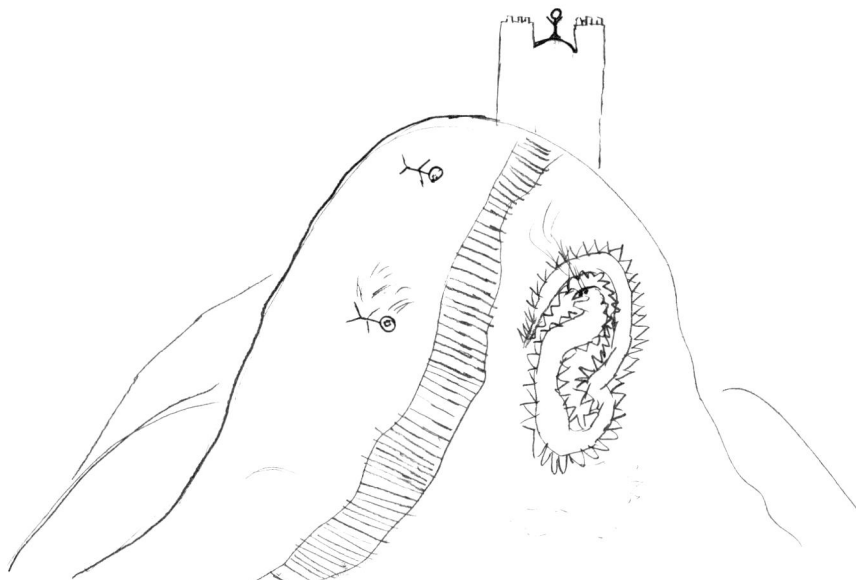

Dragons asleep in the Tor *by* Alfie

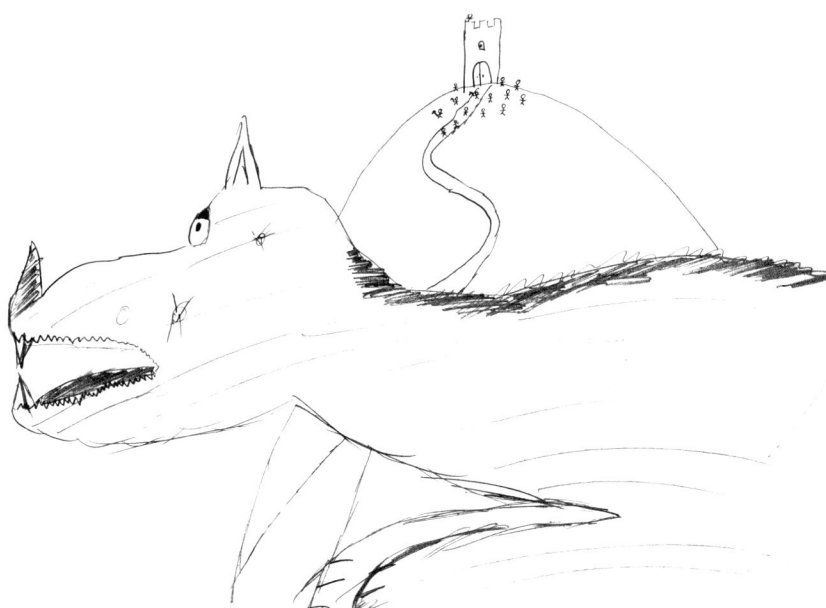

Dragons leave the Tor *by* Linden

Puppets can encourage and support storytelling and painting in educational and therapeutic settings. We have looked at large 'human' puppets with mouths that move as well as a large range of animal hand puppets that can also talk. However, for some people these puppets are too big and too overwhelming and they need something that is much smaller.

Finger Puppets

There are many finger puppets that can be purchased rather than made and some of them can form part of a 'family' with the larger hand puppets. For example there are small fox and badger finger puppets that could combine with the fox and badger hand puppets. Although these finger puppets do not move their mouths, their limbs do move and some of them can walk.

This chapter has so far been about bought puppets that can move their mouths and that both children and adults can talk through to express their thoughts and their feelings. However there are also very effective 'moving mouths' than can be made quite simply. There are simple ones made from socks described in Chapter 4. The following worksheets give further examples of human and animal puppets that can be made.

Worksheet 8.1
Simple Person Puppet

Speechmark P This page may be photocopied for instructional use only. *Creative Puppetry with Children & Adults* © Sue Jennings 2008

Side 1

You will need: three plain flexible white paper plates, scissors, stapler, pencil, ruler, 45 x 30 cms (18 inches x 12 inches) sheet of construction paper, sticky tape, scraps of material and wool.

These puppets can be 'dressed' either through painting or crayoning or by sticking on cut out shapes of clothes from material or paper. You can add hair by sticking on wool.

1 Using two of the paper plates, complete steps 1–3 of Simple Animal Puppet in Worksheet 8.2.
2 Put the paper plate puppet head on your hand as described. Place the third paper plate over the top plate half, matching the edges. It should cover the half plate (which houses your four fingers) and extend out over the back of your hand. Staple this third plate to the top half plate along the curved edges. (Make sure you are not stapling the puppet's mouth closed, and watch out for those fingers.)
3 The section of plate which extends over the back of your hand will become the upper face of the Person Mouth Puppet. Fold this section forward until it stands up off your hand. Mark a tiny 'x' on the centre of the front top edge of this plate, to indicate the top of the puppet's head.
4 On a full sheet of construction paper, draw a simple, headless human form – basically a plumped-up stick figure with two legs, two arms, simple mitten-shaped hands and a long neck. Give the body an elongated neck, about 5 or 7.5cms (2 inches or 3 inches) long. The entire body should be as tall as the length of paper allows. Cut out the headless form which will serve as the puppet's body. Prepare several of these bodies in assorted colours so the children can have a choice.
5 The top section of each paper neck should be stapled to the bottom half plate of the head at a central location next to the open edge of the thumb slot. Cover the staples with tape. The puppet body should hang down from the head. Make sure the staples and tape do not interfere with the operation of the puppet's mouth or the use of its thumb slot.

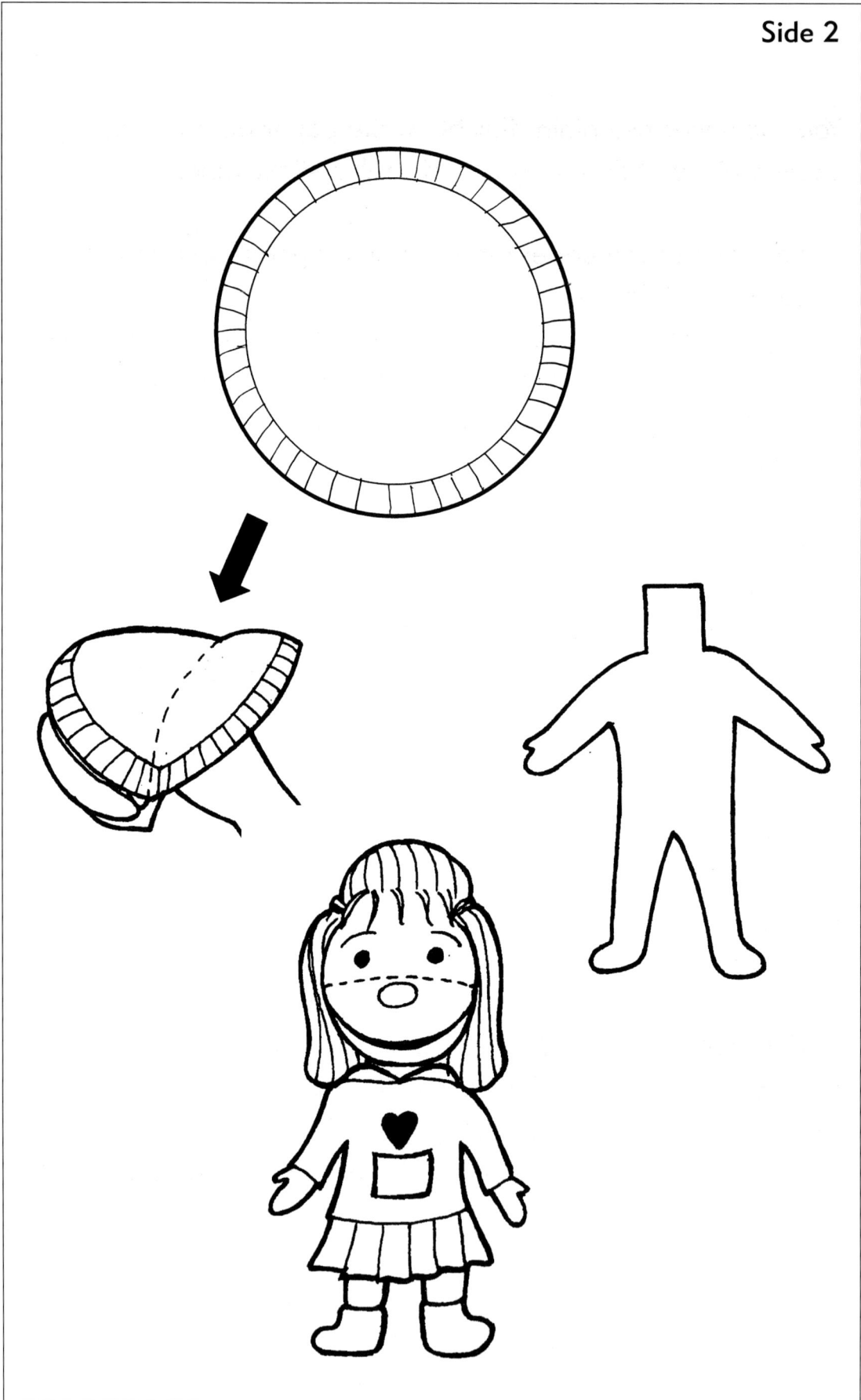

Worksheet 8.1
Simple Person Puppet

Worksheet 8.2
Simple Animal Puppet

You will need: two plain, flexible white paper plates, scissors, stapler, piece of lightweight cloth, ruler, sticky tape.

1 Fold one of the paper plates in half; open it up and cut along the fold line.

2 Lay the uncut plate bottom-up in front of you on the table. Cover this plate with the two half pieces of plate, also bottom-up, matching the edges. Staple the two plates together every 5 or 7.4cms (2 inches or 3 inches) around the outside edges of the two plates.

3 Fold the double plate in half, with the fold following along the cut lines and the plate halves and the two half-plate sections on the outside (the uncut plate will be on the inside). Slide your hand into the plate pockets, with four fingers in the top pocket and your thumb in the bottom pocket. With the plate contraption on your hand, bring your fingers toward your thumb, then away. The paper plate mouth puppet will respond by smacking its lips together in a satisfying manner.

4 Cut the cloth into a square about 30cm x 30cm (12 inches x 12 inches). You will need one cloth body for each puppet. If possible, prepare a large assortment of cloth squares in different colours and patterns, and give each child a choice.

5 Attach a square of cloth to the top plate half with staples or tape. If there are any staple prickles on the inside of the finger slot, cover them with tape for the safety and comfort of the puppeteer.

This basic puppet can be adapted to many stories; you can change the clothes, colours, hair and decorations.

Worksheet 8.2
Simple Animal Puppet

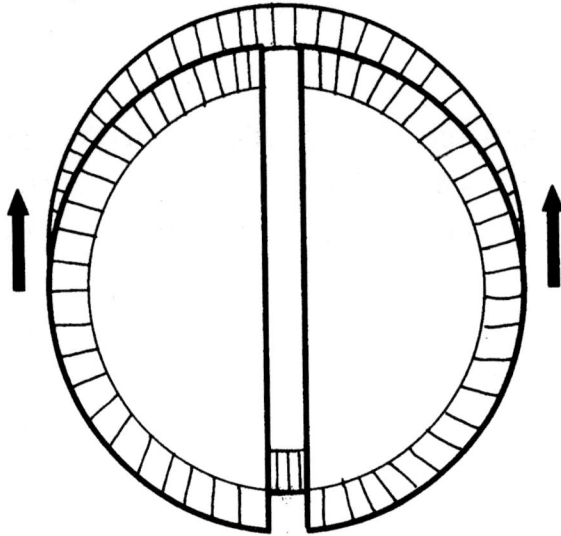

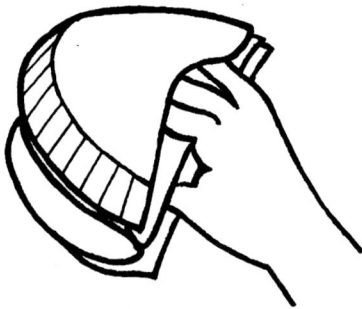

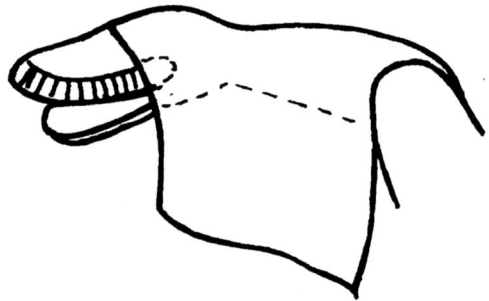

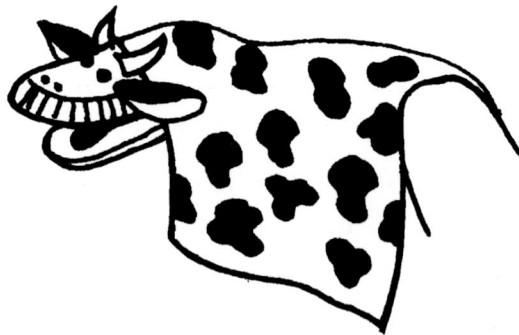

CHAPTER 9

Story Dolls: Evoking Stories

IN CHAPTER ONE I TALKED ABOUT THE DIFFERENCE between puppets and dolls, and described how a child will talk *to* a doll but will talk *through* a puppet. The exception to this usual rule is the very specific use of 'Story Dolls'. Story Dolls are especially created in order to tell stories or to evoke stories in a listening audience. The Story Doll does not move its limbs like a puppet or open or close its mouth or even move very much at all. The Story Doll can best be described as the storytellers' companion who will participate in or be a central character within a story.

There are several stories in this chapter where Story Dolls are ideal to use.

All props for storytelling, whether a puppet or a Story Doll, or a treasure box, or a magic stone, need to be treated with respect. The great tales mainly belong to ancient religions and belief systems which may or may not be adhered to in these days of technology and consumerism. Nevertheless, we need to acknowledge the power inherent in the stories or else why would they continue and be passed down the centuries? The wisdom and healing metaphors still have the power to affect us and make us think in new ways, which is why they are central to play therapy and drama therapy as well as storytelling.

The Story Doll also provides the calming element on the children for a storyteller: she or he can capture the child's attention by the doll being unusual or beautiful or eccentric. The Story Doll can introduce many aspects of storytelling and help contain the child's or group's interest and curiosity. I have a set of Story Dolls that I use both in education and in therapy. You may also decide to create a project based on children creating their own dolls and then telling a story themselves. The group may choose different stories or all be involved in the same one.

If you are working in a therapeutic setting you may decide to have a number of the Story Dolls already created and placed on a story shelf. You can invite a child or an adult to pick up and explore the dolls and see if one doll inspires a story for them. The individual can then tell you a story through the doll they have chosen. They may like you to write down their story and then tell it back to them. It may be that they choose to continue working through the Story Dolls (maybe combined with puppets), and you can put together a file or a book which contains all the stories which can then be illustrated.

You may want to choose a theme, for example 'Sea Stories', within which individuals can create their own tale of the seas. In my experience the creating of the story often happens as someone is making the doll, in complete contrast to times when I have asked someone to 'make up a story' when their minds will blank out!

Developing Literacy

Storytelling with an aide such as a Story Doll will help to develop literacy at all levels: emotional literacy, as a child is more able to express both their own feelings as well as the feelings inherent in the story; social literacy because through the storytelling they both interact with others and with the different characters in the story. And of course they will become more confident and competent in their reading and writing skills. Perhaps most importantly of all, the children will develop their 'dramatic skills' in relation to their imaginative growth, especially if their early years have been impoverished (Jennings, 2005c).

In *Creative Storytelling with Children at Risk* (Jennings, 2004) I developed an introduction to storytelling, especially through mermaid dolls. That book gives the basics in Story Doll approaches to storytelling which we can build on here.

The Making of Story Dolls

The basic principal of making Story Dolls can be adapted for different stories or themes. This pattern can form the basis for your own ideas and variations, (Royce, 2006).

Worksheets 9.1–9.3 at the end of this chapter provide you with a pattern to scale for the making of a Story Doll. These are well-tried patterns and are simple enough for most people. Do not involve the complication of joining heads, legs and arms which is a more advanced procedure – especially for children.

Making Story Dolls

The top of the doll – waist upwards – is the same for any character.

The lower half of the doll will vary depending whether you want a mermaid (see below), or

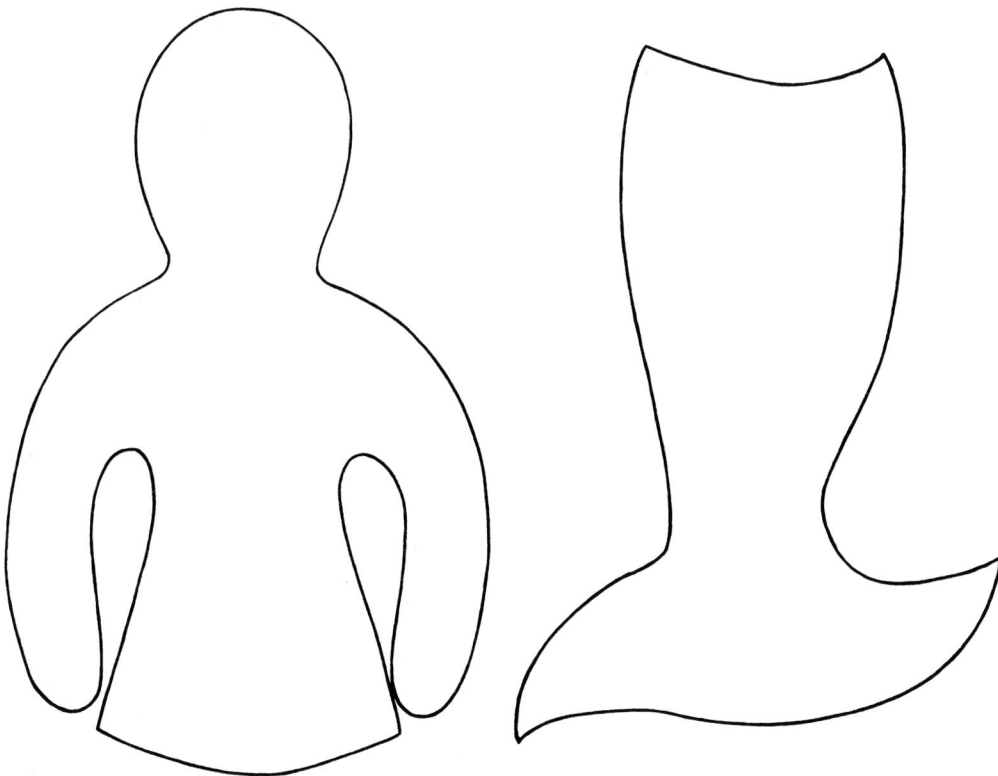

a silkie, which has a tail to the side:

or a character with legs:

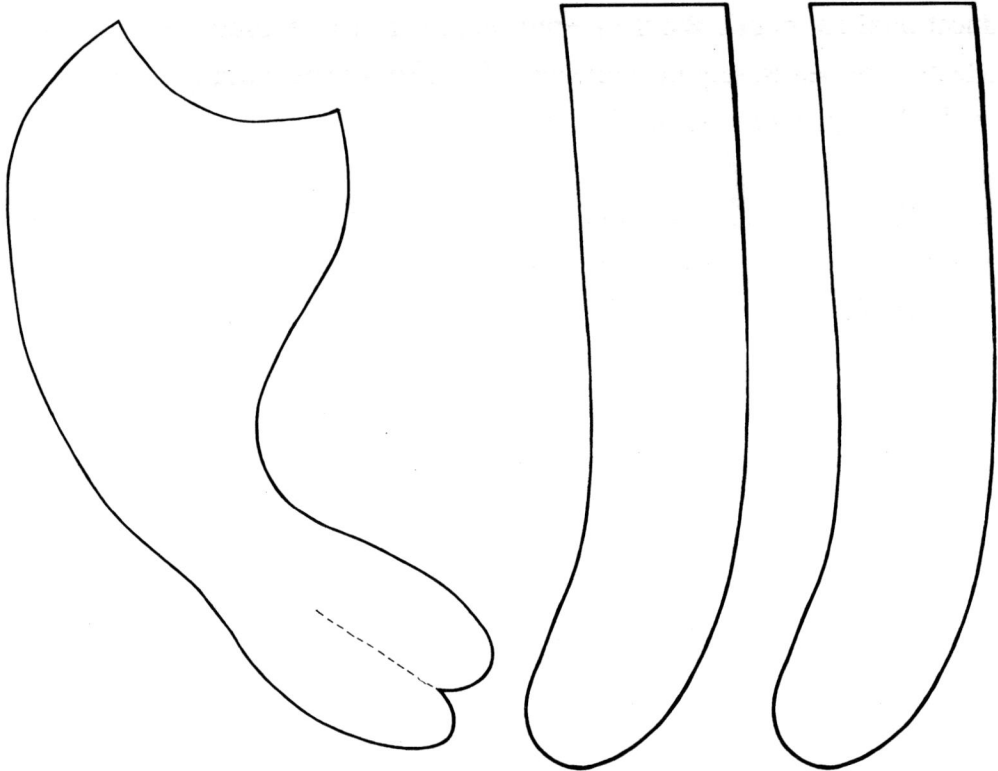

Hair, features and decorations can then be added:

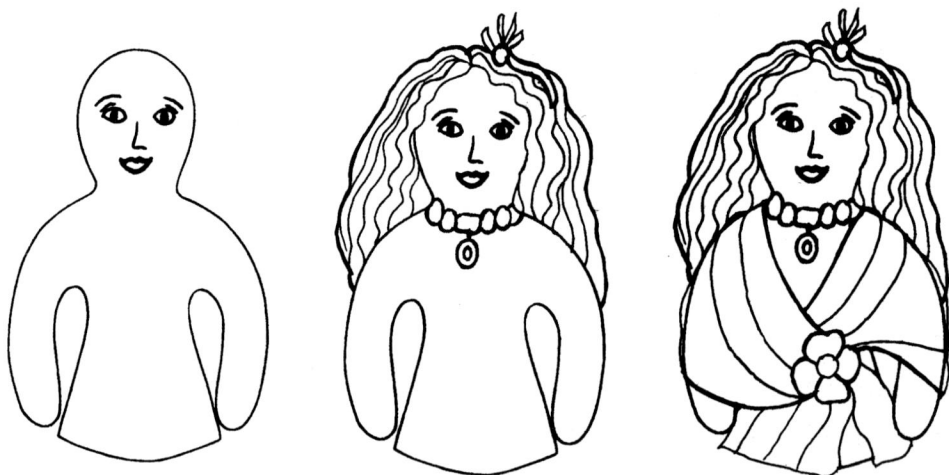

STORY DOLLS: EVOKING STORIES · **153**

You will need: Strong, finely woven cotton or polycotton to make the body; it can be plain or patterned. Stuffing that is safe, non-flammable and adheres to EU standards (or equivalent) can be bought from craft shops or educational suppliers. Wool or embroidery thread is used for the hair. A collection of beads, sequins and small decorations (depending on the age of the child) to provide the finishing touches.

Depending on the level of skill in the group you may decide to make the basic dolls in advance and then allow individuals to create the features, hair, decorations and clothes.

Elemental Dolls

The dolls that are sketched in this chapter are from my own collection that I use both in training and therapy. Mainly I choose dolls based on the elements because they yield very rich stories so I have dolls for: water, fire, earth and air.

Many of the ancient myths are based around single elements or the relationship between several elements. The elements are seen as having the power of integration and healing, and provide metaphors for exploring our inner feelings and major truths. There is always more to a story than the mere words or the beginning, middle and end. There is the story within the story and the story beneath the story, and there are symbols and images that provoke or stimulate us. The elements are among the strongest symbols for these stories.

Water Stories

Water stories can use seas, rivers and lakes, and also involve a variety of mermaids, silkies, water nymphs and sprites. The breaking of the waters heralds the birth of a new child. The crossing of water can evoke the journey to a new land and the transition into a new life or into death as we journey across the Rubicon, the Jordan or the Styx. Floods and shipwrecks are inherent in many epic tales. (The biblical story of Noah's Ark evokes probably the greatest flood of all time.) Shipwrecks herald the beginning of

Shakespeare's plays *The Tempest* and *Twelfth Night*. All these water stories could be developed through Story Dolls and indeed puppets.

The Fisherman's Story

Worksheets 9.1 and 9.2 can be used for making the silkie Story Doll and the Story Doll with legs can be used for the fisherman.

It is a long hard winter and the storms prevent many of the fishing boats setting sail. Wind is lashing up against the sea-wall and sprays over on to the rough pathway. At times the waves are so strong that they hit the window panes of the small cottages along the isolated sea front. Sometimes they are so strong that they sound like hailstones.

Although there are seven, small fishermen's cottages, only one is inhabited now, and that is the one at the end of the row, the furthest away from everything. All the other fishermen have either died or moved inland and their houses are boarded up and dark.

Jem lives alone in the end cottage and he lives for his fishing and the sea. Since his wife died he lives simply in his small house. He is happy enough; they had a good life together and shared the life of the fisher folk who lived in the other cottages. Now he has bread and a few groceries delivered each week to a metal chest at the end of the path. Every two or three weeks he walks to the village which is two miles away. He has a beer in the pub and takes any messages that have arrived for him at the post office. Sometimes if the weather is bad, then he does not walk to the village for a month or more. Very occasionally someone will walk or cycle out to see him and bring a treat – maybe an apple pie or a carrot cake.

This winter however, it is very difficult for anyone to visit anybody as the weather is so extreme and the winds are so powerful. Jem takes a stroll to the sea wall and looks out towards the horizon: there are no boats or ships to be seen and the sea looks a turbulent grey. He wanders back again and settles down to mend his nets, something that always needs doing. When it gets dark he lights a candle as he always does and places it in the window. As he dozes off in his chair he hears a light tap at the door, and again. Who on earth can be visiting at this time of night? It is very dark now and it is raining, he can hear it on the roof.

He opens he door, expecting to see someone from the village, but there is a striking looking young woman standing on his path, looking at him. He begins to say, 'And who are you…' when she smiles and says, 'I have got lost on the coastal path and now it is dark, please can you help me? It is very cold out here'. Jem starts to ask her how she has managed to stray out so far from the houses when the weather is so bad, but realises he must at least offer her shelter. 'Come in, come in,' he says, 'I will make up the fire'. She comes into his little sitting room and looks around whilst he pokes at his fire of driftwood with a few small pieces of precious coal. He turns and there she is, stretched out on his sofa, with a cloak of seal skin pulled round her. She is fast asleep!

He shakes his head and takes the candle and goes up to his tiny bedroom. He lies awake for a while listening to the wind and rain as the storm gets worse, and he wonders who this stranger is that sleeps downstairs.

The next morning there is a tap at his bedroom door and she enters and brings him a cup of black sweet tea – just as he likes it. He sits up in bed, 'Who are you?' he asks, 'I told you, I got lost in the dark and I am grateful that you sheltered me.' 'Will you tell me your name?' he asks, and she smiles almost a secret smile, and says, 'You can call me Sylvie. And you are called Jem?' He marvels that she knows his name and he wonders who she really is and enjoys the fact there is another person with whom to talk.

By the time he is downstairs, Sylvie is nowhere to be seen and he walks along the path in order to lean against the sea wall and look *out to sea. There she is standing at the water's edge and gazing into the distance across the water. She must have sensed his gaze as she looks round and smiles at him.*

'Let's go fishing,' she says. 'Get your nets ready and I will come with you'. Hm, he says to himself, the weather is unpredictable. He raises his voice and says to her, 'The weather is unpredictable, maybe we should wait?' She calls back, 'Trust me, all will be well'. He goes back to his yard and takes the nets and walks down the steep steps from the path to the narrow, shingle beach. He unties the boat and pushes it out to sea and he and Sylvie climb on board and raise the sail. The winds have dropped just enough for them to sail into deeper water. They throw the nets and she helps him pull them in, full of fish; he has not had such a big catch in ages. The wind drops completely and the boat lies still, not moving.

'We should get back,' says Jem. 'We will have to row,' and he unclips the oars and looks nervously at the sky. Sylvie takes an oar and sits beside Jem and joins in the rowing with a perfect rhythm. They arrive to the shore and they both pull the boat up the shingle and tie it securely. The storm is returning but Jem is puzzled how easily they returned, and how large the catch is today: the biggest catch he has had for many years. 'You go back to the house,' she says, 'Light the fire and I will unload the fish and put it in your fish-shed and then join you'. He is feeling strangely drowsy so he returns to the house and before he knows it he has fallen asleep on the sofa. He sleeps and sleeps right through this night and the next and awakens to a fine and sunny day.

He is puzzled that he is lying on his sofa as the sharp spring sun shines through the window. He gets up and stretches and vaguely wonders about Sylvie and goes down to the shingle. There are a few fishermen already out to sea and he goes to the fish shed and there is his great catch all gutted and dried on strings. The bigger fish are on hooks from the ceiling and all the waste is cleared away. The embers in his drying stove are quite cold so she must have finished this some time ago. He is very puzzled and as he turns there is the shadow of a figure in the doorway, 'Sylvie?' he says. 'And who is Sylvie?' asks a pleasant voice. It is Maria from the post office. 'We were beginning to worry about you, it is over two months since you have been to the village'. Jem starts to speak and then stops. He realises that she has gone back to the sea, his stranger visitor that came in from the sea. She must be one of the seal-people, not Sylvie but Silkie.

He had been cared for for the remainder of the winter because he had taken a stranger into his house that had been lost on the sea path. He smiles at Maria, 'Is that one of your apple pies?' he asks. 'Then it is time for a cup of tea.'

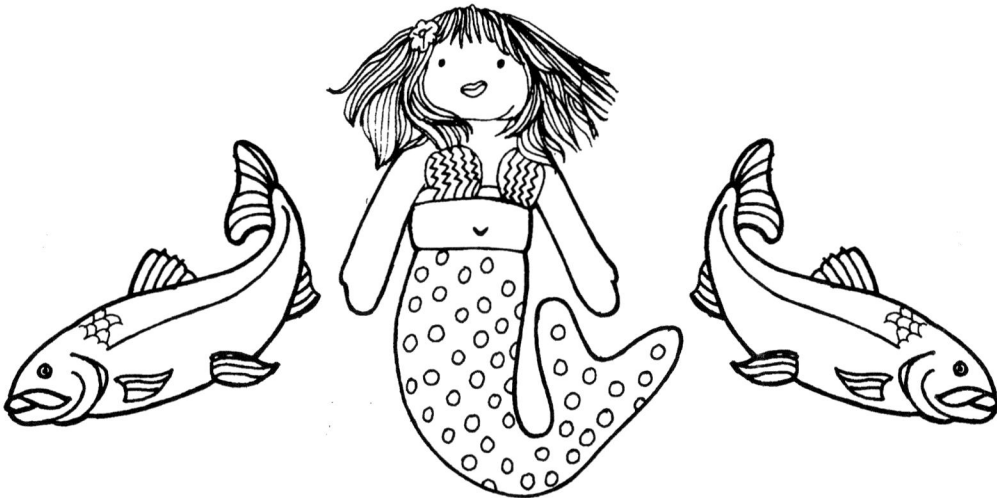

The Nine Mermaid Daughters of Atargatis
– Delphine

In *Creative Storytelling with Children at Risk* (Jennings, 2004), *Goddesses: Ancient Wisdom for Times of Change* (Jennings, 2004) and also *Creative Storytelling with Adults at Risk* (Jennings, 2005a) we told some of the stories of the nine mermaid daughters of Atargatis. In the first tale all nine mermaids follow the trader ships and arrive in Somerset and become the sprites of rivers and wells. In another story, Tara-Melusine, the sixth daughter, journeys across the ocean to the new land alone, leaving her eight sisters behind. Merlene, the eighth daughter, discovers that she has the gift of music and song and comforts an old lady in her loneliness. This is the story of the oldest sister, Delphine.

Delphine decided that she needed her own life after so many, many years of caring for her younger sisters. There were three older sisters, Delphine and Alysson and Hermione, the twins. Delphine as the first born had had a very tough life. She was the first to experience abandonment by her mother when she was left alone in the forest wondering whether anyone would come and find her. When doves came to care for her, her relief was quite overwhelming. She was loved and nurtured but rarely saw her mother, who was very busy caring for sea creatures. She was also very lonely – until that day when her twin sisters arrived. Then there were three children abandoned – they might as well have been orphans. Although Delphine felt less lonely, the twins were often wrapped up in each other and had their own secret language and private signals. Delphine felt shut out of their world at times, and she also felt responsible for them. Well, time passed, and six more children arrived; three middle children and three small children and all needed to be cared for. Delphine had to be the sensible mermaid.

One morning Delphine knows that it is time for a change: all her sisters are adult now and Tara-Melusine and Merlene have already

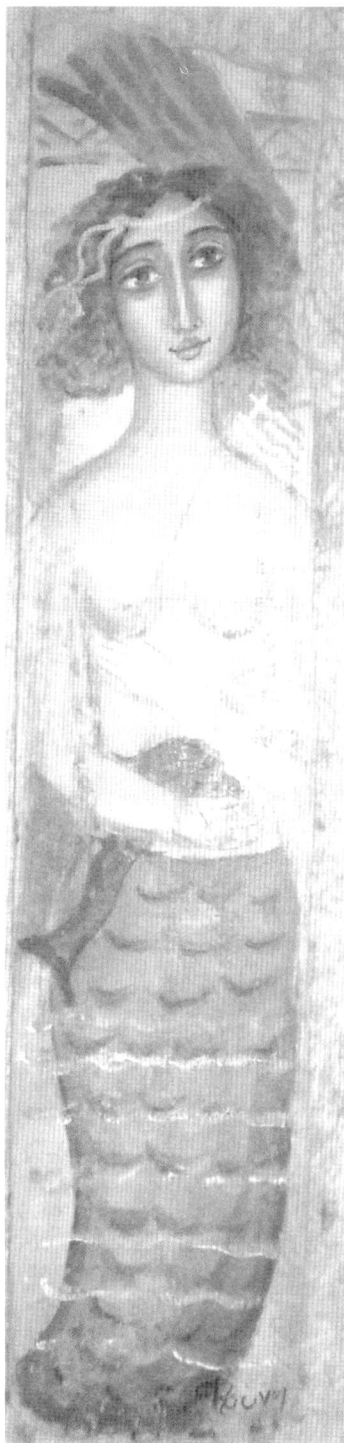

left home. But where should she go? And what could she do? She tells the twins that she needs to go away and before they can discuss it she has gone, following the coastline north, swimming with strong strokes. She arrives at the next bay and decides that she needs thinking time so she can formulate a plan. Another part of her says, 'Just go; don't plan anything.' Suddenly, she tosses her mermaid's mirror into the sea and decides to cut short her hair. These long seaweed style tresses belong to the past.

Delphine knows that she does not want to swim across the oceans like one sister and she is sure she cannot sing like another. What can she do? All she knows is taking responsibility and caring for children. All the love and affection she bestowed on them helped her too because she had been abandoned and did not know love and care.

Maybe she could do this in a new way? 'Right,' she said to herself, 'I will start a safe bay for all the mermaids who have been abandoned or orphaned. They can come here until they are adult or have been returned to their own homes. But this will be the very safe and loving home where small mermaids are wanted and loved'.

And with that she swam home to the bay and told her sisters that she would be leaving almost immediately to start a new home.

Alysson and Hermione, the Twins

The twin daughters of Atargatis had always been inseparable; Alysson was the older daughter by just two minutes. Hermione was born very quickly afterwards and they slept close to each other from the beginning. They had got over the shock of being abandoned by their mother very quickly because they had always had each other. Indeed, they could not remember a time when the other did not exist. Their older sister Delphine had mothered them and cared for them and the doves of the forest had made sure that they were safe and looked after when they were babies.

More sisters had followed on and they had helped to care for the middle sisters and the youngest ones. But no-one was more important to the twins than each other. But life is moving on and all the sisters are grown up now. Some of them have left the bay that they call home and have made new lives somewhere else.

'The other sisters have all found things that they are good at – Delphine is skilled at looking after young ones so she is going to have lots of abandoned mermaids, Tara-Melusine is the adventurer and has crossed the oceans and little Merlene found out very quickly that she can sing so beautifully,' they said to each other. 'What can we do? We are only good at watching out for each other?' They both swam and moped around the bay for a while and then they would stop and look at each other and shake their heads, 'Nothing comes to mind – nothing in my brain – what will happen?' And they swam and shook their heads again.

'Time to sleep,' they said. 'Let's talk about it again tomorrow; let's tell the story about our mum and how we were rescued by the doves in the forest'. Alysson and Hermione both stop their swimming, turn and stare at each other. They both had the same thought at the same moment, 'That's it!' they said in unison. 'We are very good at storytelling!'

They thought and thought and wondered who they could tell their stories to as up to now, for the most part, they had just told stories to each other. They remembered that sometimes they had told stories to their little sisters if they felt anxious or scared. 'Let's speak to Delphine; maybe she needs people to tell stories to her orphans,' they said. 'We can become storytellers.'

And so the twin sisters develop skills in painting pictures with their voices and encourage as many people as possible to come and listen to them. Delphine is delighted for her sisters to contribute their storytelling to her programme.

Soon the twins become renowned for their storytelling and for the first time they even dare to be apart as they tell their stories. They begin to enjoy some life apart although they are still best friends. Alysson creates and tells shadow stories which are her favourites, whereas Hermione has many star stories. When they come together they have a lot to share.

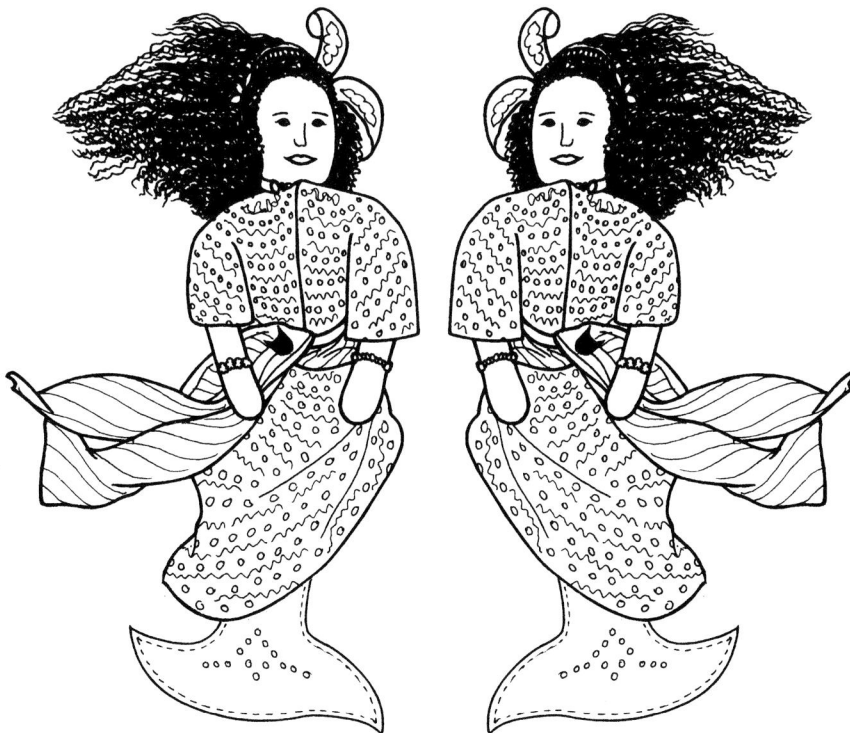

Alysson and Hermione, the twin daughters of Atargatis

Fire Stories

We have said earlier that there are many stories about fire: about discovering fire and about stealing fire and all of these can be adapted to the use of Story Dolls. The story of Pele the fire child is told in *Creative Storytelling with Children at Risk* (Jennings, 2004) and is ideal for a fire Story Doll. The doll can be made with fiery vivid colours with a skin colour of your own choosing. She can be a child, adult or old woman as the story tells of her journey through her whole life.

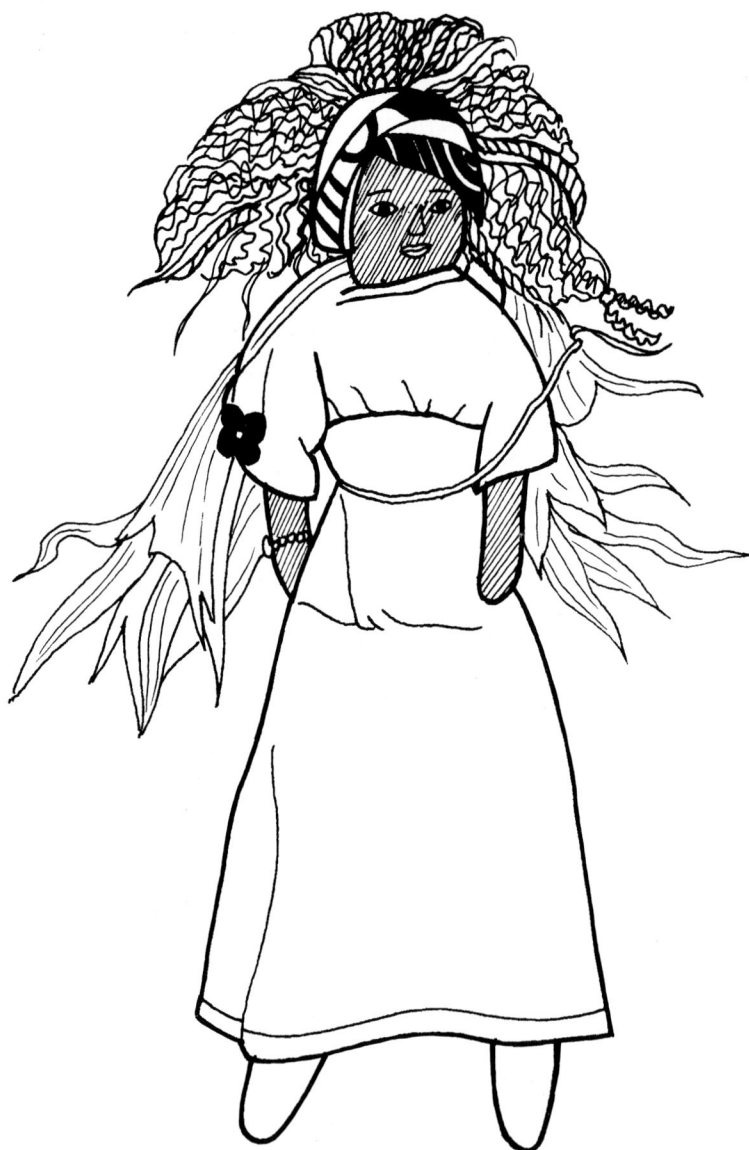

Pele, the fire child

Earth Stories

Earth tales are many and widespread and have connections with trees, with roots and growth. A doll for telling earth stories needs to have a connection with greenery and growth, perhaps inspired by the Green Man, the vegetation spirit. The great Earth Mother who is considered the oldest goddess of all, occurs in many countries: she is fertile, healing and brings growth and development. She is also firmly rooted and reaches out between the heavens and the earth. To make an earth Story Doll needs a lot of imagination and a range of materials. The temptation is to make your Story Doll too busy and therefore distract from its essential theme. (See Worksheet 9.3 for the basic Story Doll pattern.)

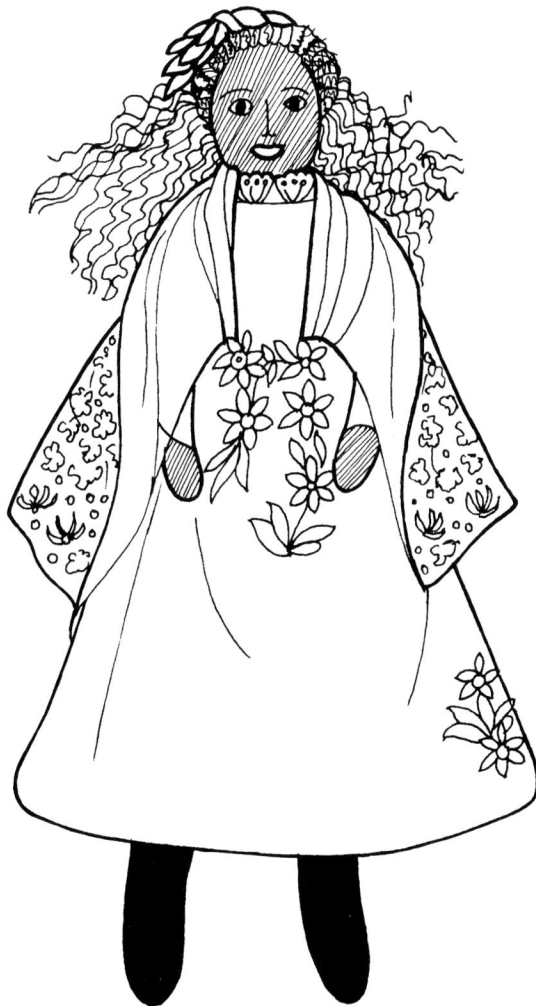

Asherah, the great goddess of the earth and trees

Air Stories

Air tales are about characters that fly through the air or feature the air itself in the form of winds and breezes. There are many stories about birds or bird people and there are also shamanic tales of air travel. Indeed, Father Christmas and his reindeer are believed to have their origin in the flying shaman. The following story about Freja can be the basis of a Story Doll and then the opportunity to create stories about love, life and death.

It is important that we are able to work with loss as well as the range of other feelings that are expressed through stories and Story Dolls. In the story about Freya and her cloak of falcon feathers we can understand Freja's grief and it will help us to understand our own. This story can also be danced and moved, painted and drawn. We can create Freja's cloak and fly through the air; we can find amber and thread our necklace, we can make her as a puppet or create her as a Story Doll.

Freja and her Cloak of Falcon Feathers

In ancient times in Scandinavia, the goddess Freja is the goddess of love and beauty, and the goddess of life and death. She is extremely beautiful and a lover of fine clothes and jewels. She is a goddess who gleams with golden colours. She wears a belt of stars, which come from Orion. She flies through the air in her chariot, which is drawn by wild ginger cats, and her long red hair flies behind her in the wind.

Freja can also fly by herself; she has a long cloak of falcon feathers and she wears it when she goes to visit the soldiers who have died in battle and have gone to the underworld. Freja is unlike many other goddesses because she is able to move between this world and the other world and can return unaided. In the underworld she invites the most handsome soldiers to feast with her at an enormous banquet. They eat off gold plates and drink from glasses cut like diamonds, and the food is plentiful and of very fine quality.

Sometimes Freja feels very sad that so many young men have to die in battles. She sits alone and stares across the battlefield, realising that she has no children of her own, and perhaps these dead soldiers are souls she can care for. She weeps quietly to herself, and large tears fall on the rock where she is sitting. As her tears drop, each one turns to amber, and there are many amber beads where she is sitting. The amber is golden like her hair and like the fur of the cats that draw her chariot, and she threads the amber onto a golden thread and wears it round her neck. She does not often cry, but when she does, her tears are golden.

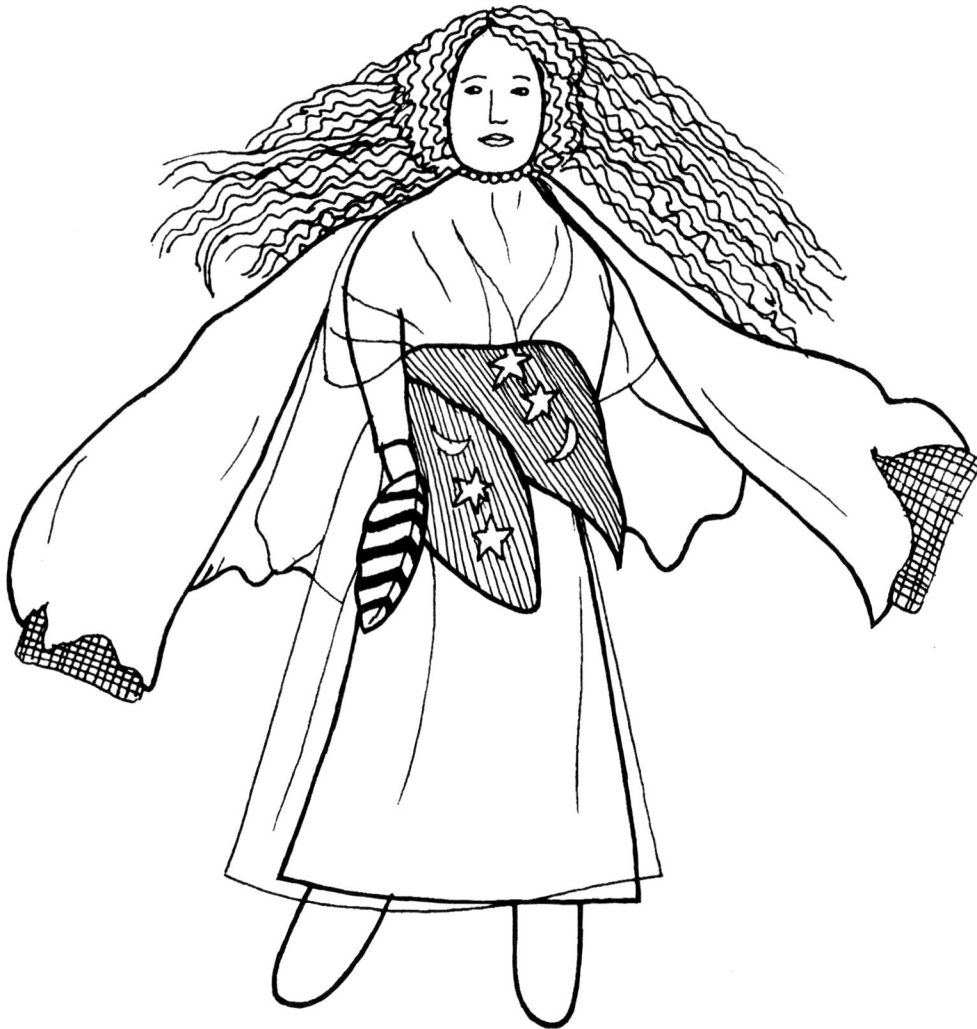

Freja, the goddess of love, life and death

Worksheet 9.1
Making a Mermaid Story Doll

Side 1

You will need: strong finely woven cotton or polycotton, stuffing that conforms to EU standards (or equivalent), wool, embroidery thread, beads, sequins, shells, ribbons, small decorations, sewing machine or needle and thread, 'soft' pencil, stick for pushing in the stuffing.

These patterns are in proportion to the Story Dolls – enlarge or reduce on the photocopier for your own purposes and allow a 12.5 mm (half inch) stitching edge.

The top of the body: cut the pattern out double, in a strong firm cotton or polycotton and machine or back-stitch along the edges shown and then turn inside out.

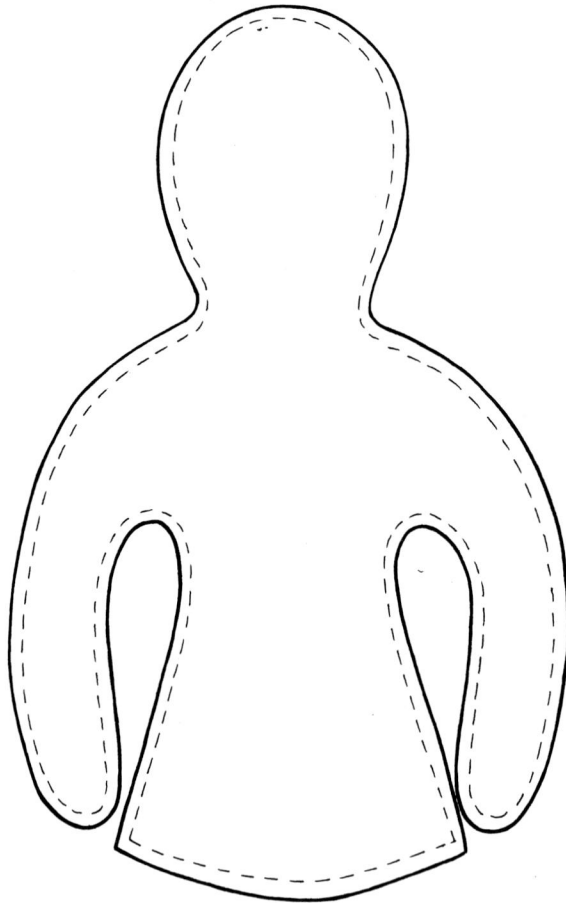

The lower half of the body: cut out the next pattern on page 167 double in a contrasting material. Machine or back-stitch it along the edges shown and turn it inside out.

Worksheet 9.1
Making a Mermaid Story Doll

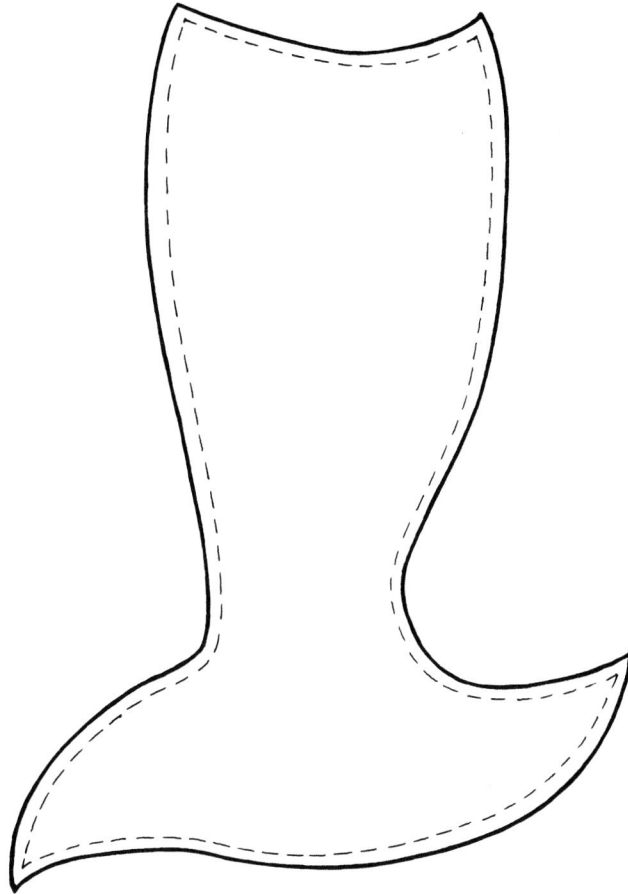

Create one small pleat in the front and two small pleats in the back. Stuff both halves with stuffing meeting EU (or equivalent) standards and then sew the two halves together, using a tacking stitch and then back-stitch on top. You may wish to embroider or sew on a belt round the waist.

Use fine wool or embroidery thread to knot the hair. Thread a needle, draw it through double and then pass the ends through the loop. Make the hair really long, then decide on the length and trim it afterwards.

Draw the features with a soft pencil and then sew them with fine cotton thread. You can stick the features on with felt, but they tend to look harsh and clown like.

You can make necklaces of tiny shells, or a pendant from a fish button or hair decorations with shell sequins. You have lots of options.

Worksheet 9.2
Making a Silkie Story Doll

Side 1

Please refer to Worksheet 9.1 for materials you will need.

Although silkies and mermaids are all from the sea, they are actually very different. Mermaids are sea creatures; half woman and half fish. Silkies are mammals and are seals that turn into humans and walk on the land. They befriend lonely humans and often live with them for periods of time but the sea always calls them back.

For the top of the silkie use the same pattern as the mermaid in Worksheet 9.1. Remember if you wish to make a bigger doll you can enlarge the pattern on the photocopier.

For the lower half of the silkie use the following pattern. The 'tails' go to the side – to right or left:

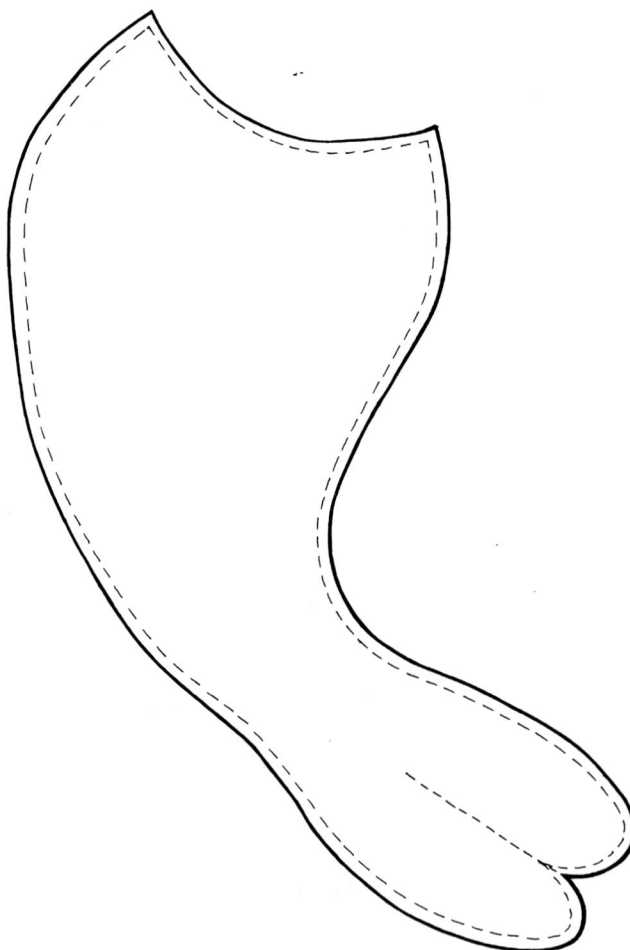

Worksheet 9.2
Making a Silkie Story Doll

Follow the same instructions for pleating and sewing for the mermaid. You may like to think of the variations for the silkie doll. Maybe the colours will vary and be more seal like. How would you create the idea of a seal skin cloak? What hair would a silkie have?

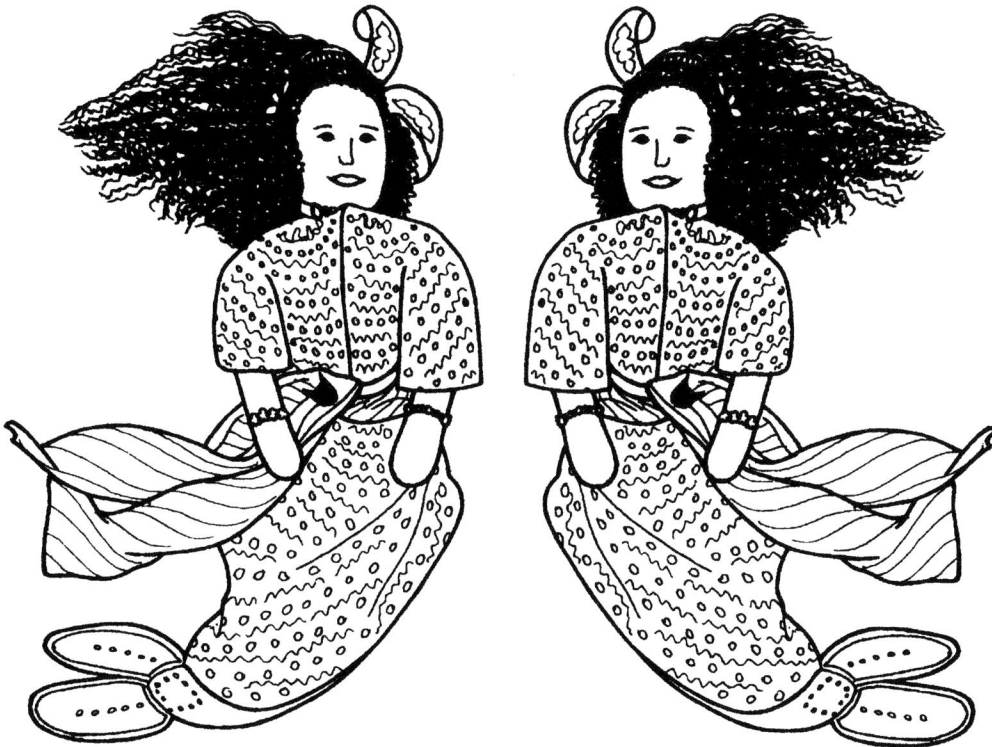

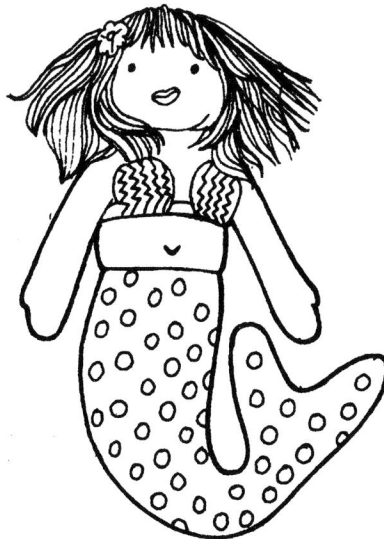

Worksheet 9.3
Making a Story Doll with Legs

Please refer to Worksheet 9.1 for materials you will need.

The Story Doll with legs rather than fins can be adapted for many different characters. You can use it for the fisherman or for the earth or air dolls, for Asherah or for Freja or characters of your own creation. The doll becomes your own individual creation with the choice of material and the hair and decorations.

The top of the doll is made from the same pattern as the previous two dolls. (See Worksheet 9.1.)

For the lower half use the 'leg pattern' and follow the same instructions for attaching at the waist. The legs need filling very carefully in order to be even rather than lumpy – you can use a cocktail stirrer or coffee stick to help it into the corners.

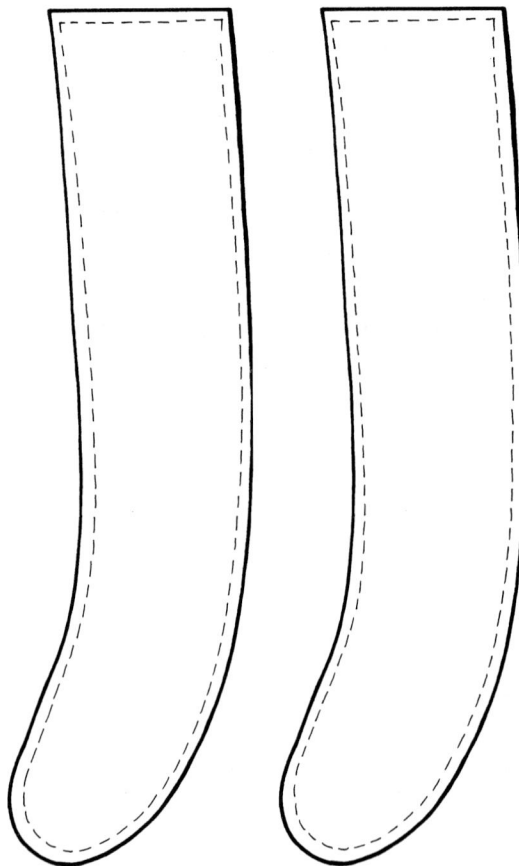

Worksheet 9.3
Making a Story Doll with Legs

Side 2

For Asherah or Freja, or your own character this doll needs a dress than can be removable or not, depending on your preference. A dress can then have a shawl or a cloak or a scarf and whatever decoration you choose. A shirt or smock for the fisherman can be embellished as you want.

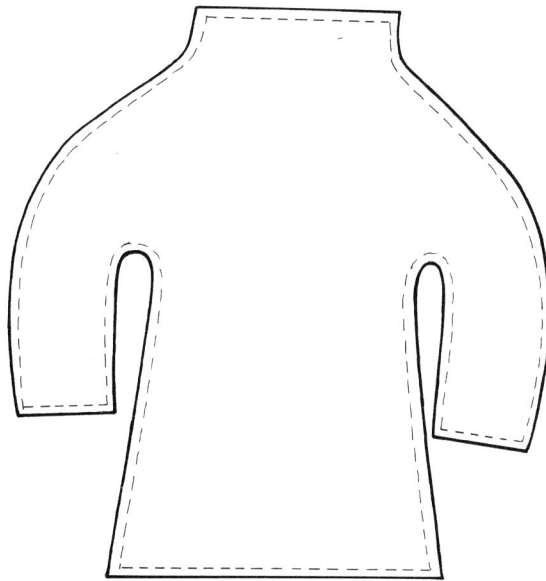

The dress can be decorated with ribbons, braid or beads, or sequins, or small feathers. Keep within the theme of the story *or* create a doll by following your imaginative impulse and see what character emerges. Then you can create your story.

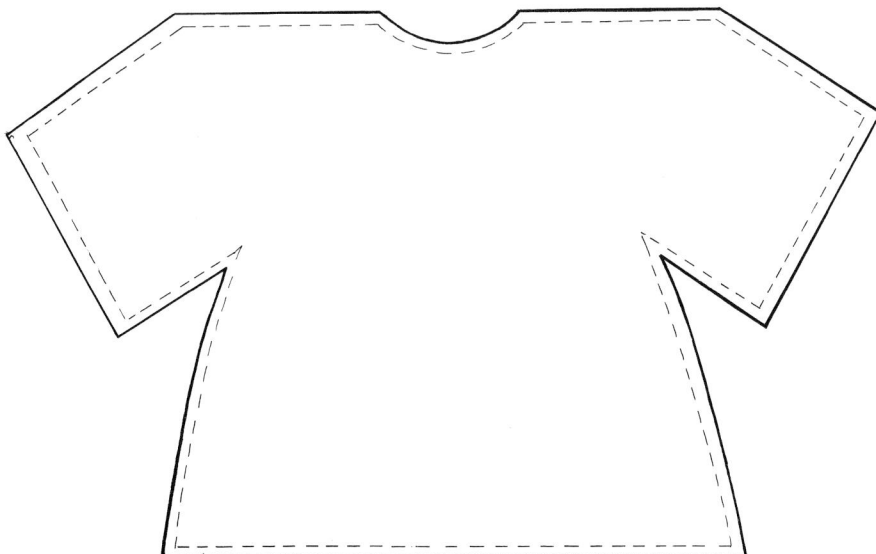

CHAPTER 10

Good Yarns for Puppets and Dolls

THIS CHAPTER OFFERS STORIES AND MYTHS that you can use to bring your puppets into life. After each story, there are suggestions about how you might adapt them and advice on possible puppets to use. However, by the time you have read the previous chapters you will already have plenty of ideas on which puppets could fit which story. These are just a few stories from the vast array of tales you might tell with puppets. You may wish to start by telling these stories and then ask the group for their ideas on developing them with puppets. There are also sources in the bibliography, including various Internet sites.

> **Remember that storytelling is an art in its own right and not just a vehicle for puppet shows! Even more importantly we need to remember that every story we tell belongs to someone's culture. Stories are precious and have special meanings, therefore we must be careful not to get into stereotypes. For example, when telling the story of how 'Coyote Helped the Karok People Steal Fire' (see below) be careful not to reproduce stereotypes of 'red Indians' with tomahawks hollering with their hands over their mouths. We can find genuine images and facts from the Internet.**

The stories themselves need to be developed with all their ideas and metaphors (Jennings, 2004b). Most puppet plays have a narrator or a chorus who introduces the story and moves the storyline on. Some of the stories you can turn into scripts: one example is the story of Red Riding Hood in Chapter 7. It may be at the beginning that you will leave more text to the narrator of the story whilst other members of the group build up their confidence and just speak a few words, if any at all, through the puppet.

Initially it may be enough to just move their puppets at the right moment. Slowly you can add sounds and then short phrases until children or adults alike are ready to take on the complete text of a character. Some groups and individuals are non-verbal and will communicate non-verbally through the movement of their puppets. People who have been involved in the making of their puppets will already be closely identified with the character and feel more confident about expressing their thoughts and feelings. They will also have ideas that have firmed through the making of the puppets. This process usually takes longer if we use a ready-made puppet and we need to leave time for 'warming up' the ideas as we can see in Chapter 2.

Remember that many people are happier doing the more technical side of drama and puppet work such as sound effects, or arranging props and scenery or any lighting effects, whereas others prefer to do a performance. For a theory of why this is so, please look back to the Introduction with examples of people's preferences based on their dramatic development, (Jennings 1998, 1999, 2005c).

When choosing a story, think about the aims of the puppet session or project. In previous chapters we looked at some of the reasons for using puppets in play therapy and drama therapy. There are also therapeutic or educational aims that are discussed in the Introduction and Chapter 1. However, it is important not to neglect the very important aims of developing the person's imagination and creativity. To be able to create through artistic media of some kind is a profound experience for children as well as adults: too often this experience is left to the 'specialist' while the rest of us have a vicarious enjoyment through watching or listening.

Societies that have traditional storytelling, folk dancing and puppet shows at the heart of their culture have their own built-in system for promoting creativity, concept formation, value systems, communication and social interaction. Stories may be told as part of their oral history as it is passed down the generations. There are family and personal stories and local community tales.

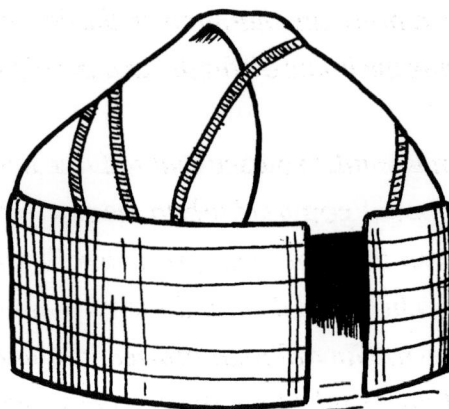

A Kazakh Yurt

How Tazsha the Orphan Outwitted a Foolish Bai

The following traditional story from Kazakhstan is typical of the many tales that recount how poor people outwit the rich or how the underdog triumphs over cruel authoritarian rulers. You can recognise some elements from the story of Oliver. Although of course we would have concerns about old men picking up young orphan boys in the market, we need to put the story within the cultural context of Kazakh folk tales and allow it to be possible that these two characters came together for companionship. As archetypes, they are the meeting of the wisdom of the old sage with the innocence of the child, and present us with symbols of integration.

The Story

In the olden days there was a young scruffy orphan who was living on the streets; indeed he was so scruffy that he was given the name Tazsha, which means scruffy or mangy! He was very bright and intelligent but was always hungry, and his hair had all fallen out.

One day he met a lonely old man in the market place. 'What are you doing here?' the old man asked. 'I am homeless and I have no family,' said Tazsha. 'Ah, you are just like me,' said the old man. 'Why don't you become my son?' And they joyously decided that they could help each other and live in peace and harmony in the little house in the woods, which became the home of Tazsha and the old man.

One day the old man said, 'You see that tall tree over there? It has a bird's nest in it. I want you to climb to the top of the tree without anyone, even the bird seeing you, and bring me one of the eggs'. Tazsha did as he was asked and quickly and carefully brought an egg down. The old man praised him and said how clever he was and then said, 'Take the egg back again just as carefully and make sure that no-one sees you'. Tazsha did just that and took the egg back again.

And so it continued this happy relationship, and Tazsha called the old man 'father' and he called the orphan 'son'. One day, the old man pointed to a house and said to Tazsha, 'In that house lives the meanest Bai you have ever met. He would not even give you some snow in winter. I think we should punish him.' 'What shall I do father?' asks Tazsha. 'Well, this man and his wife sleep with their cheeses and butter between them in sacks in case anyone steals them; I want you to creep into the house and bring the sacks to me.' Tazsha creeps into the house and easily slides out the sacks from between the sleeping couple and takes them home.

The Bai and his wife wake up and hold their heads and groan when they see what has happened. However the Bai is sure he knows who has stolen the food sacks. 'It's that scruffy orphan boy who lives with the old man in the cottage in the forest.' And he ran as fast as he could to the house and arrived there before the boy.

The Bai pretends to have the voice of the old man and says to Tazsha, 'Please go and fetch me water from the well, and give me the bundles,' and without thinking, Tazsha does just that. He returns to the house with the water and the old man is very puzzled. 'I did not ask you to get water,' he said. And immediately Tazsha knows what has happened. Tazsha rushes away to the house of the Bai and ties a white scarf around his head. 'What are you doing you old fool, don't you know that the wolf is attacking your sheep, and you disappear into thin air? Run quickly and fetch the remaining sheep safe home.' The Bai immediately does just that and drops the food sacks. Tazsha picks them up triumphantly and takes them home to the old man.

Meanwhile, the mean and foolish Bai has gone to the sheep field and found them all perfectly safe. He realises that Tazsha has tricked him and he goes home vowing to outwit him next time. But that is another story of Tazsha the clever orphan boy.

Creating a Puppet Play

This story is well suited to having a narrator and the following characters:

- Tazsha a young bald boy
- Old Man
- Bai and his wife
- possibly some sheep

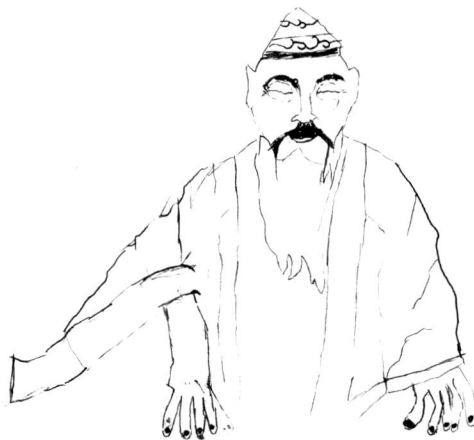

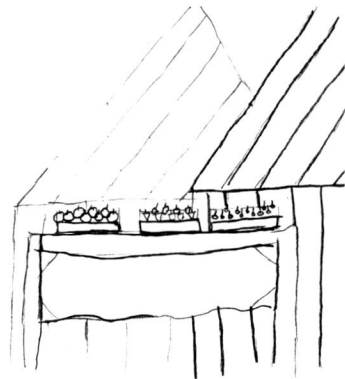

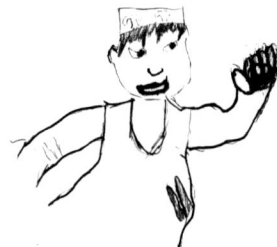

By George

Scenery

Cut-outs to represent the market where the two main characters meet (the market or 'bazaar' scene could be elaborated with different stalls and traders); the little house in the woods; the house of the Bai; most Kazakh stories have a background of mountains, horses and camels.

Sound effects: the noise of the market; Kazakh stringed music which you can find on the Internet, sheep bleating in the fields.

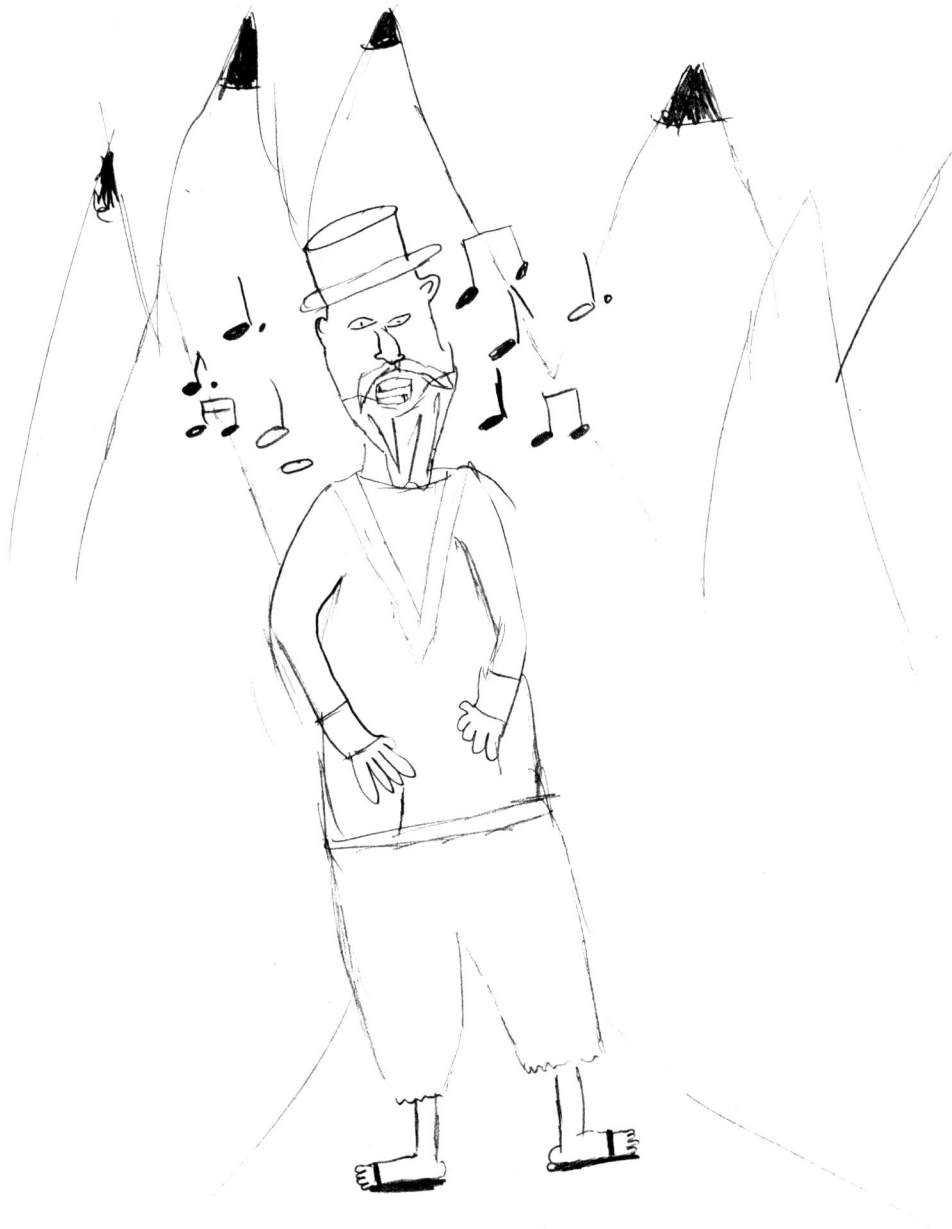

By Linden

How Coyote Helped the Karok People Get Fire

There are many stories about fire being owned by the gods and how it was stolen or obtained through trickery so that people would be able to cook and keep warm as well as making sacrifices. In *Creative Storytelling with Adults at Risk* (Jennings, 2005a), St Anthony goes to hell with his pig and cheats the devils into bringing fire back to the earth. The following story from the Karok people of North America shows how the clever coyote, a trickster animal, outwits the old hags who keep the fire, with the help of several animals and a human. It is a story of collaboration and cooperation which allows every creature to have a place, even if they do not have the most physical strength.

The Story

At this time when there is no fire anywhere on the earth, the people of the Karok tribe suffer greatly. They feel cold and miserable and see no answer to their situation. Two old hags jealously guard the fire for it is not to be given to humans. Coyote wants to help the Karok people: well, it will keep him in good standing, and he also welcomes opportunities to outwit other creatures. That is the nature of any trickster.

Coyote goes to visit the hags and slowly creeps up to their tepee, 'It's bitter cold out here,' he says in a pleading voice. 'Will you let me come and get warm by your fire?' The two hags look at each other and then say to themselves, 'He is only a coyote,' they nod and call out, 'Come in and get warm.'

Coyote creeps in and sits by the fire. Oh how warm it feels, and he looks around the tepee wondering how he can steal the fire. The two hags are guarding it and he wonders if they ever sleep. The next morning he thanks them and leaves with an idea.

Coyote calls a Great Meeting of all the animals to discuss his plan. He places creatures from the most strong to the least strong, from Lion to Frog, stretching from the Far East to the land of the Karok. There is Lion, then Grizzly Bear, then Cinnamon Bear, then Wolf, then Squirrel, then Frog.

Coyote journeys again to the tepee of the two hags, taking an Indian with him. He conceals the Indian behind the hill and goes to the tepee and calls out 'Good evening: it is bitterly cold out here, would you let me sit by your fire?'

The hags let him in to lie by the fire, saying 'He is only a coyote'. He keeps watch out of the corner of his eye and tries to plan a means of stealing the fire, and he thinks and thinks all night. The next day he goes to speak with the Indian and explains his plan. As soon as he settles in the tepee again, the Indian rushes inside and the two old hags begin to pursue him. Meanwhile Coyote seizes a fire stick and rushes away from the Far East. He gives the fire to Lion who goes running and gives it to Grizzly Bear who goes running and gives it to Cinnamon Bear; Cinnamon Bear takes the fire and goes to Wolf, and Wolf takes it to Red Squirrel who sets her tail alight and forever has a burn mark on her shoulder – you can see it to this very day. Red Squirrel takes the fire to Frog who swallows it in his big mouth; Frog cannot run so he jumps. By this time the hags catch up with them and grab Frog by his tail as he tries to jump. He jumps again and his tail comes away in their hands, which is why Frog has no tail to this very day.

Frog keeps the fire safe inside him while he swims under water until it is safe. He surfaces and spits the fire into a pile of dry brushwood and there it rests to this very day. There is always fire inside dry wood and to make it come out, the Indians rub two sticks together.

Creating a Puppet Play

You will need puppets for all the animals:

- Coyote
- Lion
- Grizzly Bear
- Cinnamon Bear
- Wolf
- Red Squirrel
- Frog

You might like to research the Native American culture and see what other animals could have been there. If you have a large group you might want to have more animals, and be sure to place them in the story, depending which animal is the stronger. As well as the animals you will need: two hags and the Indian (not a stereotype).

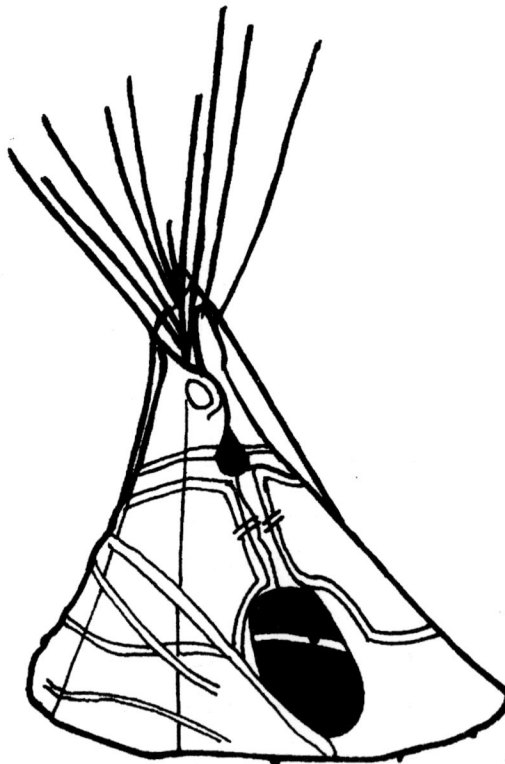

A Native American Tepee

Scenery

Create a painted backdrop of the mountains and the tepee, or you could have pieces of scenery created as 'puppet cut-outs' that can then move around. It is probably important that you have a cut-out puppet of the fire stick that can be passed from hand to hand.

Sound effects

You can also have musical sound effects such as CDs of Indian pipes and drums; you could also learn some Native American chanting.

Hansel and Gretel: a Story for Everyone

The fairy story of Hansel and Gretel is another 'into the forest' tale that is reflected in many cultures. It includes a wicked stepmother, who in some versions is the same person as the witch. This story has a strong girl who makes it possible for Hansel to escape, so that the gender balance is a little more equal!

The Story

Hansel and Gretel live with their father and stepmother in a little house a field's width away from the forest. For a while, the stepmother tolerates the children although she is never particularly friendly. However, the family is very poor and their father never has enough money to satisfy his wife's needs and she really resents the fact that the children are two hungry mouths. Eventually she persuades their father that they should abandon the children in the forest. One night Hansel is listening in to the angry conversation that his stepmother is having with his father.

He wakes up early in the morning and goes outside and fills his pocket with little white stones. He can hear his stepmother shouting for them, 'Come along you lazy children, we are going to the forest to cut wood.' As they walk along the path Hansel drops white pebbles and looks round to make sure his trail is there. 'What are you staring at you silly child?' says his stepmother.

'I am just waving to my white cat on the roof, Stepmother,' he says. 'That is not your cat,' she says. 'It is just the sunlight glinting on the white chimney.' They go to a clearing in the forest and their father lights a small fire, 'Sit here awhile while we are chopping and gathering the wood and we will call you when we are ready.' Hansel and Gretel sat and ate the small piece of bread that their stepmother had given them, comforted by the sound of the chop, chopping of the wood nearby. They dozed off and did not wake up until it is very dark.

Where is everyone?

The noise of the axe chopping is in fact a branch tied to a tree that is being blown by the wind. They have been tricked. 'Never mind, let's see if we can find the white stones to lead us home again,' says Hansel. Soon they arrive back home across the field, much to the surprise of their parents, who cover up their annoyance, especially their stepmother.

That night the stepmother makes sure they are locked in their bedroom, but even so, Hansel can hear her shouting at his father. He knows the same fate will befall them the next day but he cannot get out to gather stones. The next morning they are both given a small slice of bread then set off for the forest. Hansel drops his bread crumb by crumb. They arrive in the forest and their parents slip away. The children find the birds have eaten the breadcrumbs and they are completely lost.

They wander hither and yon until they see a little house under the trees. It is covered in sweets and gingerbread and they eagerly start to nibble. An old woman comes out of the door, 'Hello my dears, come inside, you can eat and drink as much as you wish,' she says.

The children follow her inside and there is a table covered in bread and jam, cakes and scones and juice to drink. They eat as much as they can and then lie down to sleep in the little beds. The next morning everything changes and the old woman grabs Hansel and shoves him into a cage and slams the door. 'Now my little friend, you stay in there until you get fat and chubby,' she says.

She pulls Gretel out of bed and thrusts a broom into her hand. 'You get cleaning,' she said. 'There is work to be done.' She keeps putting tit-bits of food through the bars of the cage, and each morning she asks Hansel to put out his finger so she can see how plump he is growing. He realises what she is doing so each time he puts out a chicken bone.

Meanwhile Gretel has to scrub and clean and is only given scraps of bread to eat. One morning the old woman (who of course is really a witch) says that she has waited long enough and she puts lots of wood on the fire.

'Stoke the fire for me,' she says to Gretel, 'I have cooking to do.' Gretel pretends to be very simple and says, 'Please show me what to do, I don't really understand.' 'Oh for goodness sake, it is easy enough,' she says. She opens the door of the fire and bends over, and immediately Gretel gives a huge push and the witch topples into the fire. Gretel pushes the door tight shut and the witch is left shouting and groaning in the oven.

Gretel releases Hansel out of the cage and they both take jewels and precious stones out of the witch's house. They then start to try and find their way home. There is a chirruping and a singing in front of them, and they cry out, 'It is Bluebird – now we have a guide.' The bluebird guides them through the forest for several days but soon they recognise the familiar trees near their house. They thank the bird and creep up to their house and peer through the windows. They can see their father sitting at the table looking old and sad.

They go into the house and their father hugs them over and over again and says how sorry he is. Their stepmother is dead. Hansel chides his father for being so weak and says that he and Gretel will take charge of everything. However they share the jewels with him and make plans for a happier future.

Creating a Puppet Play

This story will easily turn into a play text and you might consider creating a modern language play that could take place in the twentieth century. For example, perhaps Hansel finds his way home with his mobile phone or perhaps he and Gretel belong to Friends of the Earth and want to conserve the forest ... Let your imagine play, or even run riot!

Characters

In any case you will need puppets for the following characters

- Hansel
- Gretel
- Father
- Stepmother
- Witch
- Bluebird

Scenery

It can be relatively simple, possibly with the outline of a cottage, the field and the forest.

Sound effects

Birds of the forest, the cackle of the witch.

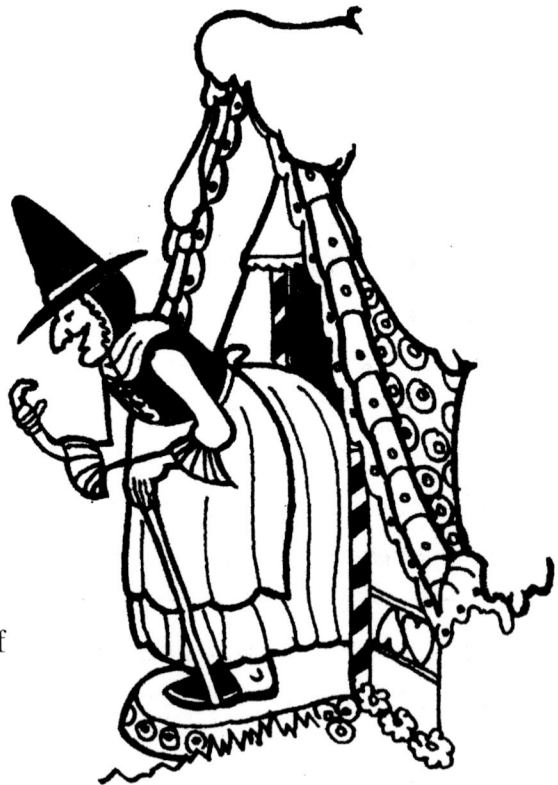

Prince Fergus and the River Monster, A Tale of Old Ireland

This is a classic story of heroes and monsters. It is also a tale of healing. It is a very sensory story, and enables people to get in touch with positive and negative sensory experiences.

High up in the mountains is a lake that is said to be very dangerous. Parents tell their children not to go near it and certainly never to drink from the water.

One day Prince Fergus and his friends are out hunting in the forest near the lake. They decide to take a rest as the weather is very hot, and they have been riding all morning. The Prince goes to drink from the lake but his friends pull him away and remind him that the lake is dangerous.

'Leave me alone,' he shouts. 'You do not really believe those silly stories.' And he takes off his jacket and jumps into the lake to cool off. The monster lying on the bottom of the lake sees the shadow of the Prince as he lies flat and floats on the surface of the lake.

The monster is enormous and has the body of a serpent and the head of a lion with rows of terrible teeth. He floats slowly towards the surface hoping to catch the Prince by surprise and devour him. However the Prince senses the movement in the water, however slight, and looks down and sees the gross creature coming towards him with teeth bared.

The Prince starts to swim for the shore and the monster is gaining on him; his great tail is whipping up a whirlpool, and the stench is overpowering. The Prince makes a superhuman effort and just reaches the sandbank in time and drags himself onto dry land, but not before the creature lashes him with his tail. When Prince Fergus arrives home his mother sees the gash on his neck, 'Where did you get that wound? You must have it cleaned, the smell is overpowering.'

No apothecary in the land was able to heal the wound. They all came with their lotions and potions but still it gaped open and still it smelt foul. No perfumier in all the land was able to create a perfume to get rid of the dreadful smell. The Prince had some special shirts made with high collars to hide the wound because soon he would be King and he must be perfect to keep that job. He did not dare take a wife because of the smell and deep in his heart he wanted to get revenge on the monster.

Then something changes; he is given a pair of magic shoes by Eisirt, the bard to King Lubdaan. The magic shoes are part of a bargain to release Lubdaan from the Irish giants. Eisirt tells him that the shoes will let him walk on water.

King Fergus tells his warriors and courtiers that he is going to challenge the monster and they try to persuade him to stay. He is determined to slay the monster, especially since it has devoured many maidens and a lot of animals in recent weeks.

Fergus stands on the shore and puts on his armour and draws his sword. He slips on the magic shoes and starts out across the lake, walking on the water. When he reaches the centre the monster rears up and creates enormous waves. Fergus and the monster go towards each other and attack, over and over again, until the lake is red with blood. The people on the shore hold their breath and do not know who the blood belongs to.

King Fergus raises his sword and plunges it into the monster and he disappears beneath the waves. The people think that all is lost. Then Fergus appears above the water again and begins to walk towards the shore, dragging the enormous head of the monster behind him. His warriors rush towards him and he leaves them to take the head while he takes off his armour and goes into the lake to wash off all the blood of the monster.

He comes out of the water realising that there is not a wound on him. The people cheer that he been such a valiant king and Fergus decides that it is time he looked for a Queen!

Creating a Puppet Play

This simple story gives the opportunity to make a more complex puppet. The sea monster can be made with several joints so that more than one person can operate it.

Characters

You will need to create puppets of:

- King Fergus
- Warriors and villagers

You might make one of his mother and involve her more in the story.

Scenery

The backdrop can represent the enormous lake and the shore, the mountain and the forest.

Sound effects

The roars of the monster and the shouts of the people will help to set the atmosphere.

So it is time to come to the end of these stories for puppets and Story Dolls. The stories can also be adapted for use with masks and drama. Stories, as we close this chapter, always bring about more stories.

The end of this whole book is really the start of your whole puppet adventure and the more you explore puppets the more involved you will become.

Not only will your groups and individual participants gain and grow from the puppets, you will also find that you change and develop in ways that you did not expect. Soon you will be able to play with puppets without referring to these stories and techniques and it will become a whole new way forward both for yourself and your work. It is important to spend time looking at the importance and significance of puppets in different cultures and how they have been adapted over the centuries to meet new social, religious and political needs. All puppets have a multi-layered function and one keeps uncovering more and more layers like a very richly coloured tapestry.

Creative Journeys!

CHAPTER 11

Useful Addresses

There are many puppet theatre and puppets organisations in the UK and overseas. Here is a selection of organisations, training centres, puppet theatres and useful suppliers. Most of the organisations have booklets and newsletters. Additional information can be found through www.google.com

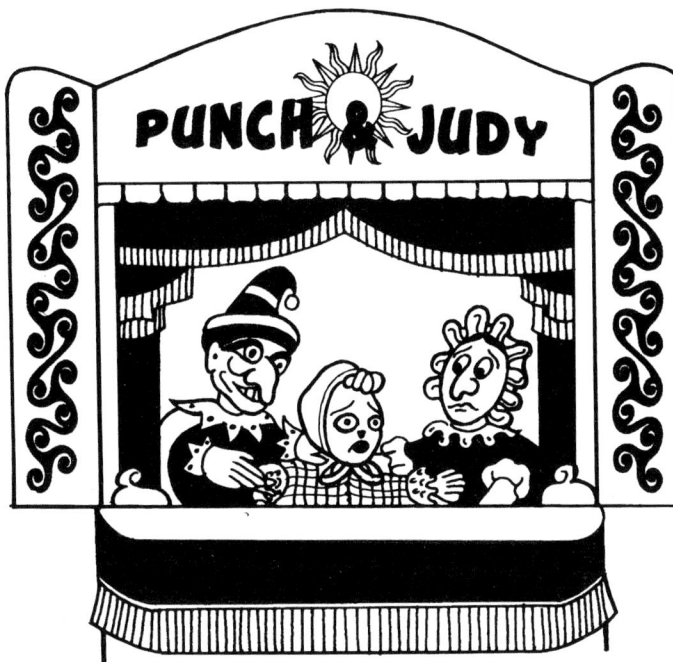

Organisations in the UK

British Puppet and Model Theatre Guild
Chair: Peter Charlton
65 Kingsley Avenue
Ealing
London
W13 OEH

+44 (0) 899 78236   peter@peterpuppet.co.uk

www.puppetguild.com

Publishes newsletter 'The Puppet Master', workshops and information.

British Centre of Union Internationale de la Marionette
Bulcamp House
Bulcamp, Halesworth
Suffolk
IP19 9LG
www.unima.org.uk

Chair: Meg Amsden
chair@unima.org.uk
+44 (0) 1502 478525

Secretary: Miriam Murtin
m.murtin@lancaster.ac.uk
+44 (0) 1524 542616

British branch of UNIMA which promotes puppetry in education and the community to promote human values such as peace and mutual understanding.

Harlequin Puppet Theatre
Rhos-on-Sea
Colwyn Bay
LL28 4EP
Webmaster: Chris Somerville
+44 (0) 1492 548166   chris@puppets.inuk.com

Punch and Judy College of Professors
www.punchandjudy.org
On-line newsletter.

World Wide Friends of Mr Punch
www.punchandjudyworld.org
Information and newsletter.

The Puppet Centre Trust
www.puppetcentre.org.uk
A library and archive open to students and researchers.

Training

London School of Puppetry
2 Legard Road
London
N5 IDE

+44 (0) 20 7359 7357   info@londonschoolofpuppetry.com

Courses for student practitioners with international specialists.

Applications for training:
The Knole
The Cross
Horsely
GL6 OPR

Puppet Theatres

Horse and Bamboo Theatre
Horse and Bamboo Centre
Waterfront
Rossendale
Lancashire

+44 (0) 1706 220241   info@horseandbamboo.org

A touring company using masks and puppets for theatres and schools.

The Little Angel Puppet Theatre
14 Dagmar Passage
London
N1 2DN

www.littleangeltheatre.com

+44 (0) 20 7226 1787   info@littleangeltheatre.com

Puppet Barge
78 Middleton Road
London
NE8 4BP
+44 (0) 20 7249 6876   puppet@movingstage.co.uk
www.puppetbarge.com
Marionettes and rod puppets, performances for children and adults.

Purves Puppets (the only puppet theatre in Scotland)
Puppet Tree House
Broughton Road
Biggar
Lanarkshire
M112 6HA
+44 (0) 1899 220631   admin@purvespuppets.com
www.purvespuppets.com
Workshops and performances.

Storybox Theatre Company
www.storyboxtheatre.co.uk
Workshops, festivals, schools.

Puppet Suppliers

Fiesta Crafts
2nd Floor
Tower House
1 Hawley Road
London
N18 3SB
+44 (0) 20 8345 6865   sales@fiestacrafts.co.uk
www.fiestacrafts.co.uk
Delightful wooden-headed finger puppets: fairy story characters,
occupations, animals and wildlife. Excellent for education and therapy.

The Puppet Company Limited
Units 204 Cam Centre
Wilbury Way
Hitchin
Hertfordshire
SG4 OTW

+44 (0) 1462 446040   info@puppetcompany.com

www.thepuppetcompany.com

A huge selection of hand and finger puppets, moving mouth animal puppets, and people. Very personal company with good understanding of education and therapy.

Puppet Book Suppliers

Ray Da Silva
58 Shreen Way
Gillingham
Dorset
SP8 4HT

+44 (0) 1747 835558   dasilva@puppetbooks.co.uk

www.puppetbooks.co.uk
www.maskandpuppetbooks.co.uk

Sacred Doll and Story Dolls
Pauline Royce

pauline.royce@hotmail.com

(No telephone number available.)

Scottish Mask and Puppet Centre

www.scottishmaskandpuppetcentre.co.uk

A specialist arts centre with studio and training workshops.

Internet Connections to the Worldwide Puppet Community

Materials, Resources & Videos

International Puppets and Therapy

www.unimalu.tripod.com

A helpful platform to use and contribute to.

Puppetry Traditions around the World

www.sagescraft.com/puppetry/traditions/index.html

An international resource linking to all aspects of puppetry.

Specialist Puppet & Mask Books

Websites specialising only in puppet and masks books, new and second hand

www.masksandpuppetbooks.co.uk

www.puppetbooks.co.uk

www.punchandjudy.co.uk

North America

ePuppets.com

PO Box 20

McCloud

CA 96057

Phone: 1-800-741-8064

Fax: 1-800-741-8064

Puppets to buy

www.sillypuppets.com

High quality products that are fun and educational.

Silly Puppets
101 W 23 Street #404
New York
NY 10011

1-800-704-5254 (Toll Free USA)
1-212-931-8542
Fax: 1-212-924-1820

info@sillypuppets.com (general enquiries)

The Feelings Company inc.
www.feelingscompany.com
Produce a variety of play therapy products.

The Small Actors Studio
Toll free in the US or Canada at: 888-880-1903
All other locations, please call: 860-599-1903
info@smallactorsstudio.com

Music
www.Bambooman.com
Bamboo music is for everybody. Listen to performances using and incorporating bamboo instruments. Buy CDs and tapes.

CHAPTER 12

Bibliography

References and Further Reading

Astell-Burt C, 2002, *I am the Story*, Human Horizon, London.

Beaumont C, 1960, *Puppets and Puppetry*, The Studio Publications, London and New York (for UNIMA).

Brooking-Payne K, 1996, *Games Children Play*, Hawthorn Press, Stroud.

Cattanach A, 1997, *Children's Stories in Play Therapy*, Jessica Kingsley, London.

Currell S, 1999, *Puppets and Puppet Theatre*, The Crowood Press, Marlborough.

Daly I, 2006, *Irish Myths and Legends*, Oxford University Press, Oxford.

Dugan EA, *Emotions in Motion*, Galerie Amrad, Montreal.

Engler L & C Fijan, 1973, *Making Puppets Come Alive: A Method of Learning and Teaching Hand Puppetry*, David and Charles, Newton Abbot.

Evans R, 2000, *Helping Children to Overcome Fear – The Healing Power of Play*, Hawthorn Press, Stroud.

Featherstone S, 2001, *The Little Book of Puppet Making*, Featherstone Education, Lutterworth.

Gerhardt S, 2004, *Why Love Matters*, Routledge, London.

Gersie A, 1991, *Storymaking in Bereavement*, Jessica Kingsley, London.

Gersie A, 1992, *Earth Tales*, Green Press, London.

Gersie A & King N, 1990, *Storymaking in Education and Therapy*, Jessica Kingsley, London.

Hansen T, 1991, *Seven for a Secret: Healing the Wounds of Sexual Abuse in Childhood*, SPCK, London.

Hathaway N, 2002, *The Friendly Guide to Mythology*, Penguin, London.

Hickson A, 1995, *Creative Action Methods in Groupwork*, Speechmark, Brackley.

Jennings S, 1986, *Creative Drama in Groupwork*, Speechmark, Brackley.

Jennings S, 1990, *Dramatherapy with Families, Groups and Individuals*, Jessica Kingsley, London.

Jennings S, 1997, *Playtherapy with Children: A Practitioner's Guide*, Blackwell Science, Oxford.

Jennings S, 1998, *Introduction to Dramatherapy: Ariadne's Ball of Thread*, Jessica Kingsley, London.

Jennings S, 1999, *Introduction to Developmental Playtherapy: Playing for Health*, Jessica Kingsley, London.

Jennings S, 2000, *Brigid: Fertility, Creativity and Healing*, Rowan Studio, Wells.

Jennings S, 2001, *Inanna: Journey into Darkness and Light*, Rowan Studio, Wells.

Jennings S, 2003, 'EPR – A Model for Dramatic Play', in *Play Words*, April/May.

Jennings S, 2004a, *Creative Storytelling with Children at Risk*, Speechmark, Brackley.

Jennings S, 2004b, *Goddesses: Ancient Wisdom in Times of Change*, Hay House, London and San Francisco.

Jennings S, 2005a, *Creative Storytelling with Adults at Risk*, Speechmark, Brackley.

Jennings S, 2005b, *Creative Play and Drama with Adults at Risk*, Speechmark, Brackley.

Jennings S, 2005c, *Creative Play with Children at Risk*, Speechmark, Brackley.

Jennings S, 2006, 'Creative Ageing', in *Journal of Nursing and Residential Care*, January.

Jennings S, 2006, *Storytelling and Play in Kazakhstan*, DVD Actionwork, Bleaden.

Jennings S, in press, *Creative Play and Stories with Babies at Risk*.

Jennings S & Hickson A, 2002, 'Pause for Thought: Action or Stillness with Young People', in *Communicating with Children and Adolescents*, A Bannister & A Huntingdon eds, Jessica Kingsley, London.

Jennings S & Minde A, 1993, *Art Therapy and Dramatherapy: Masks of the Soul*, Jessica Kingsley, London.

John M, 2001, *Children's Rights and Power*, Jessica Kingsley, London.

Kalff D, 1980, *Sandplay: A Psychotherapeutic Approach to the Psyche*, Sigo Press, Santa Monica, CA.

Lahad M, 2000, *Creative Supervision*, Jessica Kingsley, London.

Latshaw G, 1978, *The Complete Book of Puppetry*, Dover Publications, New York.

Lowenfeld M, 1935, *Play in Childhood*, Mackeith Press, London.

Malik J, undated, *The Puppet Theatre of the Modern World: an International Presentation in Word and Picture*, Harrap, London (for UNIMA).

Marshall HE, 1907, *Stories of Roland Told to the Children*, TC & EC Jack, London (currently published by Yesterday's Classics, Chapel Hill, NC).

Mellon N, 2000, *Storytelling with Children*, Hawthorn Press, Stroud.

Meyer R, 2001, *The Wisdom of Fairy Tales*, Floris Books, Edinburgh.

Moyles JR, 1989, *Just Playing? The Role and Status of Play in Early Childhood Education*, Open University Press, Maidenhead.

Newham P, 1999, *Using Voice and Theatre in Therapy*, Jessica Kingsley, London.

Oaklander V, 1978, *Windows to our Children*, Real People Press, UT.

Royce P, 2006, Personal communication.

Rump N, 1996, *Puppets and Masks: Stagecraft and Storytelling*, Davis Publications, Worcester, MA.

Scott M, 2005, *Irish Folk and Fairy Tales Omnibus*, Time Warner, London.

Sherborne V, 2001, *Developmental Movement for Children*, Worth Reading, London.

Slade P, 1954, *Child Drama*, Hodder & Stoughton, London.

Slade P, 1995, *Child Play: Its Importance for Human Development*, Jessica Kingsley, London.

Stoppard T, 1976, *If You're Glad, I'll Be Frank*, Faber & Faber, London & Boston.

Further Reading

THE BOOKS IN THIS LIST give a comprehensive overview of working with puppets in many different media and throughout the world. They are classics in the field and may take some resourcefulness to locate!

Bernier M & J O'Hare, *Puppetry in Education and Therapy, Unlocking Doors to The Mind and Heart*, AuthorHouse, Bloomington, IN.

Bauer C, 1997, *Leading Kids to Books through Puppets*, American Library Association, Chicago, IL.

Benegal S, 1960, *Puppet Theatre around the World – India*, Caxton Press, ID.

Brecht S, 1988, *The Bread and Puppet Theatre*, Methuen, London.

Champlin C, 1980, *Puppetry and Creative Dramatics in Storytelling*, Nancy Renfro Studios, Austin, TX.

Chaney C, *Plaster Mould and Model Making*, Prentice Hall, New York.

Dagan EA, *Emotions in Motion. Puppets and Masks of Black Africa*, Galerie Amrad African Art Publications, Montreal.

Efimova N, 1935, *Adventures of a Russian Puppet Theatre*, Puppetry Imprints, Birmingham, MI.

Ewart FG, 1988, *Let the Shadows Speak – Developing Children's Language Through Shadow Puppetry*, Trentham Books, Stoke-on-Trent.

Hobart A, 1988, *Dancing Shadows of Bali: Theatre and Myth*, Kegan Paul, London.

Hunt T & N Renfro, 1982, *Puppetry in Early Childhood Education*, Nancy Renfro Studios, Austin, TX.

Jenkins PD, 1980, *The Magic of Puppetry. A Guide for those working with children*, Prentice Hall, New York.

Jurkowski H & P Francis, 1966, *History of European Puppetry from its Origins to the end of the 19th Century*, Mellen Press, Lewiston, NY.

Law JM, 1997, *Puppets of Nostalgia. The Life, Death and Rebirth of the Japanese Awaji Ningyo tradition*, Princeton University Press, Princeton, MA.

Luomala K, 1984, *Hula Ki'i, Hawaiian Puppetry*, Institute for Polynesian Studies.

Muhlmann SL, 1988, *Music for the Puppet Theatre*, Dover Publications, New York.

Matusky PA, 1994, *Malaysian Shadow Play and Music*. SE Asian Monographs.

Mazzacane MS, *Music Education Through Puppetry*, Keynote Publishers, London.

Painter WM, 1989, *Musical Story Hours. Using Music with Storytelling and Puppetry*, Library Professional Publications.

Renfro N, 1979, *Puppetry and the Art of Story Creation*, Tools for Schools.

Renfro N, 1984, *Puppetry, Language and The Special Child*, Nancy Renfro Studios, Austin, TX.

Roth CD, 1975, *The Art of Making Puppets and Marionettes*, Chilton Book Company, USA.

Rump N, 1995, *Puppets and Masks. Stagecraft and Storytelling*, Davis Publications Inc, Worcester, MA.

Stalberg RH, 1984, *China's Puppets*, China Books & Periodicals.

Thurston J, 1996, *The Prop Builder's Molding and Casting Handbook*, Betterway Publications.

Van Schuyver J, 1993, *Storytelling Made Easy with Puppets*, Greenwood Press, Westport, CT.

Wills WH & LM Dunn, *Marionettes Masks and Shadows*, Doubleday Doran & Co., New York.

Warshawsky G, 1985, *Creative Puppets for Jewish Kids*, Behrman House Publishing, Springfield, NJ.

Zurbeche MS, 1987, *The Language of Balinese Shadow Theater*, Princeton University Press, Princeton, MA.